Remodelling Hospitals and Health Professions in Europe

Other recent titles also by Mike Dent

MANAGING PROFESSIONAL IDENTITIES: Knowledge, Performativity and the 'New' Professional (co-editor – Stephen Whitehead)

GENDER AND THE PUBLIC SECTOR (co-editors – Jim Barry and Maggie O'Neill)

Remodelling Hospitals and Health Professions in Europe

Medicine, Nursing and the State

Mike Dent
Professor of Health Care Organisation
Staffordshire University

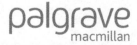

First published 2003 by
PALGRAVE MACMILLAN
Houndmills, Basingstoke, Hampshire RG21 6XS and
175 Fifth Avenue, New York, N.Y. 10010
Companies and representatives throughout the world

PALGRAVE MACMILLAN is the global academic imprint of the Palgrave Macmillan division of St. Martin's Press, LLC and of Palgrave Macmillan Ltd. Macmillan® is a registered trademark in the United States, United Kingdom and other countries. Palgrave is a registered trademark in the European Union and other countries.

ISBN 0–333–76067–0 hardback

This book is printed on paper suitable for recycling and made from fully managed and sustained forest sources.

A catalogue record for this book is available from the British Library.

Library of Congress Cataloging-in-Publication Data
Dent, Mike, 1944–
   Remodelling hospitals and health professions in Europe : medicine, nursing, and the state Mike Dent.
      p. cm.
   Includes bibliographical references and index.
   ISBN 0–333–76067–0
   1. Medical care—Europe.   2. Nursing—Europe.   3. Social medicine—Europe.   I. Title.

   RA395.E84M556 2003
   362.1'094—dc21
                                                        2003048275

10   9   8   7   6   5   4   3   2   1
12   11   10   09   08   07   06   05   04   03

Printed and bound in Great Britain by
Antony Rowe Ltd, Chippenham and Eastbourne

Contents

List of Figures and Box

Figures

Box

Glossary of Foreign Terms, Abbreviations and Acronyms

Dutch

AVVV – General Assembly of Nursing and Allied Health Professional Groups.

CBO National Organisation for Peer Review in Hospitals.

KNMG – Royal Dutch Medical Association

LCVV – National Centre for Nursing and Care – a federation of professional nursing and care providers funded by the government.

Maatschappelijk middenveld – the 'middle field' where the government has some power as well as responsibility for balancing out the claims of the various interest groups in order to represent a consociational public interest – approximating to a national interest.

maatschappen – the independent partnerships of hospital specialists. A form unique to the Netherlands.

Nieuwe Unie – NU'91 – National Nurses Association of the Netherlands.

NIVEL – The Netherlands Institute for Primary Health Care.

NIZW – The Institute for Care and Welfare.

NZI – National Hospital Institute.

VERVE – Society of Nursing Scientists.

verzuiling – 'pillarisation' of society. This peculiarly Dutch institutional arrangement formally established in the early part of the twentieth century has effectively enabled Catholics, Protestants and secularist interests to co-exist within a coalition of social solidarity.

Wet BIG – Individual Health Care Professions Act.

French

Agence Nationale Pour le Développemment de l'Evaluation Médicale (ANDEM) – National agency for the development of medical guidelines and evaluation.

ANAES (*Agence Nationale d'Accreditation et d'Evaluation*) – Nationale Agency for Accreditation and Evaluation responsible for accreditation across the public and independent sectors.

Association Française des Infirmiéres Diplômés et Élèves (ANFIIDE) – Association of French Nurses – The main organisation for public sector hospital nurses established 1924

Assurance-Maladie – the statutory health insurance – sickness fund – system.

Brevet de Capacité Professionel – Nursing Certificate and legal qualification to practice.

cadres supérieurs infirmiers, the nursing managers at ward level.

Caisse National d'Assurance Maladie des Travailleurs Salariés (CNMATS) – the National Sickness Fund, which is under state control.

Caisses Primaires d'Assurance Maladie – Primary Sickness Funds.

Caisses Régionale d'Assurance Maladie – Regional Sickness Funds.

carte sanitaire – 'health map' of 200 geographical health sectors for determining health needs and provision of hospitals and clinics.

chef de service – head (chief) doctor of a hospital speciality or service with responsibility to provide medical leadership.

Conféderation des Sydicats Médicaux Français (CSMF) – Confederation of Medical Unions of France

Confédération Français démocratique du travail (CFDT) – Democratic union for white-collar and technical workers (historically a Catholic union)

Confédération générale du travail-Force ouvrière (CGT-FO) – General union of industrial workers/working class (historically the communist union for manual workers).

directeur des soins – director of care.

droits – rights

étatisme and *étatiste* – highly centralised state organisation, particularly associated with France.

Fédération des Médecins de France (FMF) – Federation of the Physicians of France.

Fédération des Sydicats Médicaux de France (FSMF) – Federation of the Medical Unions of France.

hôpital-entreprise – Hospital enterprise.

infirmier anesthésiste – anaesthetic nurse

infirmier de bloc opératoire – theatre nurse,

Infirmier Generale – Director of Nursing – literally Nurse General

infirmier – title of nurse

l'Ordre des Médecins – The Order of Medicine.

la médecine libérale – the principles of the relationship between the independent medical practitioners, the sickness funds and the state.

Médecins Généralistes France (MG France) – Union for medical generalists

médicin référent – general practitioner or independent medical generalist.

medico-technique – clinical and laboratory services

mutualles – private insurance to cover the cost of official co-payments for health care.

Programme Assurance Qualite (PAQ) – Programme for Quality Assurance in hospitals based more on TQM (Total Quality Management) principles than directly with clinical practice.

Programme Hospitalier de Recherché Clinique (PHRC) – programme for clinical research in hospitals.

puéricultrice – paediatric nurse

Références Médicales Opposables (RMOs) – Medical or clinical guidelines/ protocols.

Regime General – the largest sickness fund scheme, which covers 80 per cent of the population.

réhabilitatition – allied health professions

Sécurité Sociale – Social security

service infirmier – nursing specialty.

Société Royale de Médecine – Royal Society of Medicine existed prior to the French Revolution, established 1778.

Societes Savantes Savants – medical associations.

Syndicat National des Cadres Hospitaliers (SNCH) – union of hospital directors.

syndicats – trade unions.

ticket moderateur – the co-payment component of the patient's health care costs.

Union des Syndicats Médecaux Francais (USMF) Union of the Medical Unions of France.

volonté général – Rousseau's principle of the 'general will'.

German

gesetzlich – legal, lawful.

Allgemeines Krankenhaus – German public sector hospitals.

Ärztekammern 'Doctors' Chambers', the local medical professional association (*Ärztekammer*: singular).

Ärztetag – Federal Doctors' Chamber i.e. all Germany.

Assistenzärzte is a qualified doctors approximately equivalent to specialist registrars in the UK

Bund – federal (i.e. national) level.

Bundesrat – the upper house of the German parliament , which has the power to overturn legislation from the *Bundestag* (the lower house).

Bundesstaat – federal state i.e. the German state

Chefärzte – Chief doctor of a hospital specialty.

Deutsche Gesellschaft – German scientific association or society.

Deutscher Berufsverband für Pflegeberufe (DBfK) – German Nursing Association

Erfüllungsgehilfe – willing instrument or servant.

Ersatzkassen are alternatives (substitute funds) to the German statutory health insurance open to white collar and technical workers.

Fallgewichte – relative weight.

Fallpauschalen – 'case fees' i.e cost per surgical case and a precursor to the introduction of DRG (Diagnosis Related Groups) costings.

Fortschritt – Progress

gemeinschaft – community.

Gesetzliche Krankenversicherung (GKV) the German statutory health insurance.

Gesundheits-Struktur-Gesetz – the Health Care Structure Law, 1992.

Grundgesetz – Basic Law of the German constitution

Hamburg Krankenhausgessellschaft – the Hamburg association of hospitals.

Krankenhausgessellschaft – the State Hospital Association.

Kammer – chamber (singular)

Kammern – chambers (plural)

Land – state (singular)

Länder – states (plural)

Landesbetrieb Krankenhauser (LBK) State Enterprise Hospitals, the public sector hospital corporation, for Hamburg

Landtag – state government (Germany comprises of 16 states)

Marburgerbund is the union for hospital doctors.

Mitteleuropean – central European

Oberärzte senior physician one level below *Chefärzte*.

Rechtsstaat is a term used to define a state (and its public administrative system) that is based on – and legitimised – by a legal system and formally recognised rights in contrast to the Anglo-Saxon concept of 'public interest' (Pollitt and Bouckaert 2000: 53). The emphasis on 'rights' (*recht*) is a characteristic of all corporatist welfare regimes.

Sonderentgelte – 'procedure fees' relating to surgery and a precursor to the introduction of DRG (Diagnosis Related Groups) costings.

Stationsärzt is an *Assistenzärzte* responsible for the day-to-day patient care on a particular ward

Teamarbeit – Teamwork

Vivantes, the public sector hospital corporation for Berlin

Wahlleistungspatient – 'paying patients' i.e. private patients within a public hospital.

Greek

Eleftherotypia – *Freepress* – a Greek newspaper.

Enosis Iatron Nosileftirion, Athinon-Piraeus (EINAP) – Union of Hospital Physicians.

EΣY – National Health System of Greece.

fakelakia – means 'little envelopes' the illicit informal payments made by patients and their families to physicians, and especially surgeons in expectation of more attention and better care.

IKA – sickness fund for industrial workers – manual and non-manual.

KEΣY – Central Health Council.

OGA – sickness fund for rural workers (who make up over half the population). It is funded wholly by the state.

Panellionios Iatrikos Sillogos (PIS) – Pan Hellenic (Greek) Medical Society.

PASOK – Pan Hellenic Socialist Party.

Sillogos Epistimonikou Igionomikou Prosopikou (IKA) – Society of Professional Health Personnel of IKA or SEIPIKA

TEVE – sickness fund for small businesses and merchants.

Italian

Azienda Ospedaliera – public hospital enterprise similar to a hospital trust in the UK.

Aziende Sanitarie Locali – local health enterprises/authorities.

collegi – colleges, the regulatory body for occupations that require only college diploma entry (*college*, singular form).

Compromesso Storico – the 'historic compromise' when in the 1970s the Communist party joined the governing coalition with Christian Democrats.

dirigente medico di primo livello – first-level physician

dirigente medico di seconda livello – second-level physician.

l'Olivo government – Centre Left and Green coalition – in power late 1990s until 2001.

La Questione Meridionale – 'Southern Question' which refers to the problems of economic and industrial development and political corruption in Southern Italy.

laurea – a university degree.

Legge Bassanini – the law (*legge*) of the early 1990s that significantly extended powers to the Italian regions.

Mansionerio – list of nursing duties prescribed under the law.

ordini are the state regulatory bodies (orders) for the professions (*ordine*, singular form). Graduate (*laurea*) entry.

Partitocrazia – rule by political parties i.e. social and career advancement only possible under the patronage or sponsorship of political parties.

Servizio Sanitario Nazionale (SSN) – National Health Service.

tangentopoli- 'bribesville' a popular description of the widespread corrupt political practices in Italy prior to the 1990s.

unitarie sanitari locali (USL) – local health units providing primary care, outpatient services and social services.

Polish

Gminas – directly elected town and village councils which are beginning to replace the ZOZ (see below) in the administration of primary and community care.

Izba Lekarska – Doctors' Chambers, similar to the German *Ärztekammer*.

Polska Zjednoczona Partia Robotnicza (PZPR) – Polish Trade Union of Health Workers' Party.

Polskie Towarzystwo Lekarskie – Polish Physicians' Association, a scientific association.

Powiats – local government, which has been re-created and is becoming increasingly responsible for the district hospitals replacing the centralised ZOZ system (see below) of health administration.

Sejm – the Polish parliament.

Semashko – the Soviet model found throughout Eastern and Central Europe, a strongly centralised system of health care delivery that concentrated resources on acute, specialist hospitals.

Voivodship – regional state – an administrative region not autonomous federal state.

Zespol Opieki Zdrowotnej (ZOZ) health management units, part of the communist centralised bureaucracy that continued to function as the health care bureaucracy well after the collapse of the communist regime.

Zwiazek Zawodowy Lekarzy Polskich (ZZLP) – Trade Union of Polish Physicians.

Swedish

Arbetarrörelsons Efterkrigsprogram (1944) – *Post-war Programme of the Workers' Movement* known also as: *The Twenty Seven Points* (*De 27 Punkterna*).

Hälso-och Sjukvärdens Ansvarsnämnd – Medical Responsibility Board.

kronor – Swedish currency = 'crown'

Landsorganisationen i Sverige – the national union organisation.

Landstingsförbundet – Federation of County Councils.

legitimerad sjuköterska – newly qualified nurse.

Medicinalstyrelsen – National Board of Health until 1968.

Medicinska Kvalitetsrådet – Medical Quality Council (MQC), a joint body established by the SMA and SSM.

Nationella riktlinjer – National Guidelines established under the Dagmar-agreement of 1996.

omvårdnad – nursing.

polikliniks or *primärvården* – outpatients, or ambulatory, clinics.

Riksdag – Parliament.

röntgensjukoterska – radiology nursing.

SDP – Social Democratic Party

Sjukhusläkarföreningen – Swedish Association of Hospital Physicians previously known as *Overläkarföreningen*.

Socialstyrelsen – National Board of Health and Welfare (NBHW) came into being in 1968 following the merger of National Board of Health (*Medicalstyrelsen*) and the National Board of Social Affairs (*Socialstyrelsen*).

SPRI – Swedish Institute for Health Service Development.

Svenska läkaresällskapet – Swedish Society of Medicine (SSM), a scientific society.

Sveriges läkarförbund – Swedish medical association (SMA) the doctors' trade union, representing well over 90 per cent of the doctors.

Acknowledgements

The work on which this book is based could not have been carried out without some serious help. Each country and hospitals visited was made possible with the generous help of a great many people. They are thanked here in the order that I visited each country. The first country visited outside the UK was The Netherlands where it was Ruud van Herk, then based at Erasmus University, who invited me across and gave me a place to stay. Sweden was next on the itinerary and here it was Hans Hasselbladh, then of the University of Stockholm, who organised the research access. The Polish research came about as the result of meeting up with Ken Khoudry (UCSD, San Diego) and Dick Raspa (Wayne University) at the Standing Conference of Organisational Symbolism meeting in Warsaw in 1997. My second trip to Poland a year later was made possible principally with the help of Adrian Szumski, Academy of Entrepreneurship and Management, Warsaw whose help with the logistics of accommodation, transport and interpretation was invaluable. Gerard de Pouvourville (IMAGE, Paris) organised the research access in two hospitals in France and gave up much of his time too in order to ensure all went well. Professor Aris Sissouras and Nikos Fakiolas (National Centre for Social Research) provided me with introductions and office space, and one of them gave me a memorable ride around Athens on the back of his moped. My second visit to Greece was organised with the very successful help of Minas Samatas (University of Crete). The Italian component of the research was the most comprehensive, due to the amazing abilities of George France of the National Research Institute, Rome. Finally, without the help and imagination of Chris Howorth (Royal Holloway, University of London) and Claudia Preuschoft (Café Real, Hamburg) there would not have been a German case included in this study, as the original plans fell apart. As for the UK it is not possible to name anyone as that would breach the necessary rule of anonymity, but there are some persons to whom I do owe and acknowledge a sizeable debt of gratitude. There are others too who have given much crucial help either in the organisation of field trips or in later discussion around the writing of this book. These were, in alphabetical order: Jim Barry (University of East London); Elisabeth Berg (University of Lulea); Marc Berg (Erasmus University); Maria Blomgren (Uppsala University); Viola Burau (Brunel University);

Jeff Butler (Public Health, Berlin); Peter Garpenby (Linkoping University); Maggie O'Neill (Staffordshire University); Maria Petsemalides (University of Thrace); Jonathan Pratsche (University College, Dublin); Jane Salvage (editor of *Nursing Times*); Rita Scheppers (University of Leuven); Robyn Thomas (University of Cardiff); Marcin Wojnar (Warsaw Medical School).

I must also record my thanks to all the doctors, nurses, managers and others who gave of their time freely, many of whom were immensely helpful to me. The fact that they all remain anonymous does not lessen the gratitude.

The research would not have happened without the financial support of Staffordshire University Research Initiative Funding and, in the final stages, that of the School of Health, Staffordshire University. I also need to acknowledge Sage Publications for permission to reproduce an amended figure from the *Journal of European Social Policy* as Figure 2.2 as well as Elsevier Science for permission to reproduce a figure from *Social Science & Medicine* as Figure 3.1.

Finally, I acknowledge that all the mistakes are my very own.

1
Reorganising Hospital Medicine and Nursing in Europe

It will not have escaped the notice of anybody who happens to be living in Europe at this time that the organisation of health care services has been and continues to be in a seemingly permanent state of flux. In some countries this is perhaps more noticeable than others, but no health system is free of the challenge of change. The dynamic for this process has been primarily, but not solely, one of controlling costs, but the modernising of health services delivery within Europe has proved to be not simply one of financial stringencies. Coping with the cost implications of the raised expectations of the citizenry and of new medical and related technologies at the same time as trying to control rising public expenditure levels generally has meant governments attempting to change the rules of the game and not only finding new ways of funding health care but also trying to reconfigure the social and cultural expectations of the users and the professionals. This first chapter sets the scene for the more elaborate analysis in Chapter 2 and the series of four comparative case studies to follow.

The changing policy context

A useful starting point is McGregor's (1999) 'three ways for social policy in late capitalist societies'. This article relates specifically to the UK; nevertheless it does provide a preliminary schema with which to locate a discussion of the European varieties of the Welfare State, not because it suggests a 'fits one, fits all' solution but because it provides a way into a discussion as to how European states choose to differ in their approach to health service reforms. The analysis is not restricted to health but addresses the issue of social policy generally and argues that there are three tendencies within advanced capitalist societies:

1

1   welfare state
2   neo-liberal regime
3   paternalistic social state or 'third way'.

These are not so much alternatives to one another but seemingly exist on a time line. The first, the Welfare State, lasted from around 1945 to the mid 1980s. The second, neo-liberalism, shared the limelight with the Thatcherism and Reaganism of the 1980s and it is still with us despite it waning in influence and giving way to a 'new paternalism' of the 'third way' associated with centre-left governments, especially 'New Labour' in the UK.[1] Within the broader European context the concept of 'new paternalism' is an intriguing one because, first, it raises the possibility that there is an alternative to a neo-liberal future for the Anglo-Saxon world and, second, it seems to suggest that there may be the possibility of a convergence between the paternalistic social state and either the Conservative corporatism of much of continental Europe or the Social Democratic Scandinavian model rather than the usual assumption that neo-liberalism is the only show in town. It is these possibilities that will be examined within this book.

The form which European paternalism takes varies between the unitary and federal states even if the consequences appear similar (Pollitt and Bouckaert 2000:41). To take a key issue of this book: the implications of health care reforms for the medical and nursing professions. Under the Welfare State model of the second half of the twentieth century the professions, and especially the medical profession, dominated. Neo-liberalism, with its emphasis on the centrality of the market, undermined this professional dominance. In principle, health professions, including hospital specialists, became skilled labour power to be managed by a new cadre of managers according to new principles of public management. The paternalistic social state (or 'third way') continues to subordinate the professionalism to managerialism, but the principles within health care are now more focused on 'managed care' than 'marketisation'. Within the 'managed care' discourse all the welfare regimes of Europe can engage, for the model does not appear to challenge their underlying assumptions in the way that narrowly defined neo-liberal solutions have done.

Reforming health care systems

It is perhaps surprising how little account UK policy analysts, politicians and the public appear to take of other European systems of health care organisation and reforms. This is certainly the case when compared to the attention given to North America. There are in many ways good reasons for the Anglo-Saxon orientation of much UK policy and organisational analyses in addition to the convenience of a common language. The common traditions, similar legal systems and cultural expectations, at least to some extent, would explain this. Possibly more compelling is the fact that the USA has acted as a massive laboratory for social experiment for much of its existence, not least in health care (Kirkman-Liff 1997:39–40; Moran 1999:173). This has not necessarily been to the benefit of US citizens, who in the case of health care have suffered greatly in the cause of liberty and market freedoms. Many are underinsured and un- or under-cared for while the system as a whole is the most expensive in the Western world. But for Europe, and particularly the UK, it has provided a constant source of inspiration for reform and thinking through the paradigm shift that produced the health maintenance organisation and, more generically, 'managed care' (Scott *et al.* 2000:40–4) which would appear to have become the touchstone for health care reforms that are still continuing across much of Europe although they began back in the 1980s masked by a neo-liberal rhetoric of regulated markets and competition in The Netherlands, UK and Sweden.

From the 1980s the organisation of health care across Europe began to undergo major changes and these have had important consequences for medicine and nursing as well as for patients and their families. Initially the reforms were driven by the rationale of 'quasi-markets' (that is, regulated or internal markets), especially in the UK and Scandinavia, but during the 1990s this gave way to a more managerialist agenda increasingly referred to as New Public Management (NPM) (Hood 1995). The impact of this paradigm within Europe has been variable but discernible, first, because the administrations within several countries within continental Europe were resistant to its siren appeal, preferring instead to rely on making adjustments to pre-existing corporate frameworks. Second, the adoption of NPM has been introduced as a means of reforming pre-existing organisational arrangements resulting in distinctive national or regional variants. Third, the division of labour, professional organisation and jurisdiction (Abbott 1988) of hospital doctors and nurses also vary across European countries. This is largely a reflection of the welfare regimes (Esping-Anderson 1990) but also mirrors social and cultural relations of different societies, not least those relating to family and gender. This book is about how all of this is reflected in the range and forms of medical autonomy and dominance across Europe, as well as the implications they have for nursing and its professionalisation, and the consequences for public management reforms of health care services. There is much that would suggest there has been a convergence in the organisation of health care across Europe partly driven by European Union (EU) regulations and partly from the secular impact of New Public Management (NPM), which in health care shares some common characteristics with managed care (Fairfield *et al.* 1997; Ranade 1998:6–8) and partly by the increasing globalisation of health and medical technologies. The most significant driver for any putative convergence, however, has been the pressure to contain costs.

European health care systems have all been seriously challenged by the cost implications of ageing populations and technological developments (Kanavos and McKee 1998:24), a concern amplified by the challenge of globalisation. Governments have tended to be concerned by escalating costs of public sector healthcare because of the belief that it will undermine their international competitiveness. In the process, older assumptions of citizenship and the Welfare State (Marshall 1950) have suffered a major 'legitimation crisis' (Habermas 1976), a consequence, in part, of the economic crisis of monopoly capitalism and consequent rationality crisis of the administrative arrangements of the Welfare State. Esping-Andersen (1996:2) suggests that the problems are related to the failure (but not the impossibility) of welfare states to adapt to the new socio-economic order. The attack of the neo-liberals on European welfare states has effectively undermined the older assumptions. But ideology on its own would be insufficient to have caused the rupture with the past had it not been for the 'new global economy... [that] mercilessly punishes profligate governments and uncompetitive economies' (ibid.).

The question of convergence of European health care services is a complex one, and while there is a growing similarity in the philosophy behind the reforms the organisational principles and practice may remain different (Saltman 1997) and convergence may be a myth although possibly a useful one (Pollitt 2001). The argument that will be presented here is – while accepting the potency of the forces for convergence – there are other deeply embedded social and cultural as well as political forces that resist, adapt or undermine managerial reforms and which reflect the reality of specific countries' health systems (see also Jacobs 1998). The relations between nursing, medicine, the public and the state are strongly shaped by such forces, which while certainly not immutable, nevertheless impose a strong 'magnetic' influence on attempts at reforms. They are particularly influential in relation to the boundaries between public/private health care provision and the gendered construction of much of health care work, especially nursing. The particular concern here is to examine the ramifications of organisational reforms and cost containment policies for medicine and nursing and their interrelations. This is as an exercise in the comparative analysis of health care organisations combined with the sociology of professions and involves adopting a meso-level organisational sociology perspective within a macro-level comparative framework (Mohan 1996), one that draws on Esping-Andersen's (1990) template for analysing welfare regimes. In more concrete terms, the book describes the professional and organisational changes of medicine and nursing in relation to management within acute hospitals across Europe. The reason for this focus can be succinctly stated. The acute hospital occupies a central and dominant position within virtually all the European health services despite a range of pressures to shift the emphasis more to primary care and general practice. Such a shift, it is widely assumed, would improve the general health of the population as well as being more economic with resources than hospital-based care (for example, Stevens 2001:160). Yet it remains the case that the acute hospital and the physicians working within it continue to enjoy a high status at the apex of the health care system. This is the place where the leading specialists may be found, where the most advanced technology is located, and a place that is often one of local pride. The focusing on acute hospitals, along with hospital specialists and nurses, is not the result of any myopia regarding wider changes in primary care, community-based services or the contribution being made in certain countries of health promotion and prevention. Rather it reflects the continuing ascendancy of the acute hospital within health care systems regardless of those developments and in part sustained by patient preferences. It would appear that wherever patients have the choice they prefer to consult specialists rather than generalists even if their condition does not warrant it. In fact it is only where the general practitioner is formally established as the gatekeeper to secondary care, as in the UK, that this practice is suppressed or driven out of the public sector into the private. Where reforms in the primary sector and public health have proved to be effective they do impact on the numbers of acute hospitals and change their role and status within the broader health service landscape. As will become clear in later chapters, however, there is a substantial degree of inertia within the health systems of many countries that has inhibited any radical disestablishment of hospitals in favour of primary and community care.

The organisation of the book and selection of countries

The chapters of this book are organised according the following rationale. The issue of the relation between welfare regimes and health systems is discussed in Chapter 2, which also provides an overview of the European health care systems, their hospital organisation and that of the medical and nursing professions too. It is this chapter that sets out the extended argument of this book. It starts with a review of the range and variation of European welfare regimes and sets out in a preliminary way the implications this has had for the professional organisation of nurses and doctors. Having set out the welfare regime context, the chapter then focuses on health systems and hospital organisation. The task here will be to assess the relevance or otherwise of New Public Management (NPM) to hospital organisation and across Europe. Finally, and deriving from the earlier discussions, a theoretical framework is constructed, one that draws on new institutionalism (Powell and DiMaggio 1991; Scott *et al.* 2000), although not in an uncritical way.

The following four chapters comprise the paired case studies. Eight countries have been selected as examples of the different regions and systems within Europe. These countries have been paired in order to strengthen the comparative element of the analysis, with each chapter focusing on themes particularly relevant to those countries as well as providing a general description of the health care system and the professional organisation of medicine and nursing. This is a selective approach that does mean certain aspects of a particular country's health system and/or medical and nursing organisation may be understated or possibly ignored. It would always be difficult to provide a definitive account of each country as that would require a book on each. Equally, I wished to avoid the repetition of revisiting themes at length across every chapter. Nevertheless, it is intended that the themes raised in the earlier case studies are reflected or taken up in the later ones, for example the issue of professional accountability is treated in the first case study comparison (Chapter 3): and is discussed to some degree in each of the later studies. The selected pairing of countries in chapter order is as follows:

- The Netherlands and Sweden
- UK and France
- Germany and Italy
- Poland and Greece.

The selection of countries and their pairing reflects a rationale provided by Pickvance (1999:355) that 'comparison requires (a) commensurability (rather than similarity), and (b) the construction of theoretical models linking contextual features to the main relationship of interest'.

The main themes treated within these comparative case study chapters are as follows: professional accountability and governance (Netherlands and Sweden); state–professions relations and governmentality (France and the UK); regionalism versus federalism and the implications for medical and nursing organisation and work (Germany and Italy); the role of clientelism and familialism within the Polish and Greek health services. The theme of subsidiarity is also one that permeates most chapters, for it links community (*gemeinschaft*) and state within the corporatist regimes and appears to promise an alternative way of integrating health care services in the others. It was Esping-Andersen's (1990) model of welfare regimes that provided the initial guideline for selection but there were other considerations taken into account as well. The selection includes both larger and smaller countries (in terms of population) as well as examples of the corporate, social democratic and putatively '(neo-)liberal' varieties. The fourth pairing (Poland and Greece) represent examples of transitional and southern European regimes not included in Esping-Anderson's original typology. The issues of professional autonomy and medical dominance run through all the chapters, while the phenomena of clientelism haunts much of the discussion too.

In the final chapter the argument of the book is restated and the strands of professional autonomy, social and cultural embeddedness, and the state are brought together and the implications of any managerial reforms for medicine, nursing and hospitals organisations are summarised.

A note on the methods of inquiry

This comparative study was started in the mid 1990s and is based on literature research coupled with field trips to each of the countries.[2] The main focus of the latter was initially the hospital doctors and their professional organisations, with management and nursing playing a secondary role, a function of the limited resources of time as much as funding. The rationale for the research visits to each country was that they enabled me to check out my understanding and interpretation of the English language literature and provide new leads with which to interrogate the literature further. It is not my intention here to make any rigorous methodological claims, for the account presented in this book is neither solely, nor predominantly, based on these field trips and interviews. What they do offer, however, is additional information and illustrative materials as well as evidence to cross-check some of the findings reported in the secondary literature.

There was already an extensive literature on European new managerialism and health policy (for example, Altenstetter and Björkman 1997; Pollitt and Bouckaert 2000) as well as on the medical profession (for example, Johnson, Larkin and Saks 1995) although some of the more interesting analyses are within more general accounts of the European professions (Abbott 1988; Krause 1996) and country-specific texts (for example, Wilsford 1991; Knox 1993) and in journals. But in the case of the nursing profession in Europe there is relatively little English language literature. Yet it became increasingly clear to me that nursing was not to be ignored, for the issues and challenges facing nurses were part of the same dynamics that were affecting medicine, and to ignore the profession would be to miss out a crucial part of the account.

Concluding remarks

This book brings together organisational, sociological and policy analyses of health care organisations and professions in order to provide a comparative study of changing hospital organisation, medicine and nursing across Europe. It also examines the future of the professions as a mode of occupational organisation within the public sector and the changes in terms of jurisdictions and boundaries between them (that is, medicine and nursing) and within the state, civic culture and civil society. These are analysed with reference to concepts of familialism, subsidiarity and clientelism, and the implications these have for the gendered construction of professionalism and legitimacy of professional autonomy. More generally my intent has been to critically assess the overgeneralisation of 'convergence' and seek out differences and the reasons for them. The picture that will emerge is one of a range of networks of professional, managerial, political and lay actors configured according to historical and social conditions as much as by cost considerations, although cost containment policies do appear to be the prime mover for policy change. The ways of understanding the dynamics of these networks as a basis for comparative analysis is set out in the next chapter.

2
European Hospitals, Medicine, Nursing and Management

The purpose of this chapter is to present the theoretical framework underlying the accounts presented in the following chapters. The chapter is in three parts, beginning with an examination of the European Welfare State regimes (Esping-Andersen 1990). The middle section moves the focus from the regimes to the professions, with an analysis of medicine and nursing. This involves an assessment of Weberian and Marxian approaches to the sociology of the professions. In the final part the focus shifts from health professions to health care organisations, with a discussion on European public sector management reforms which will draw on the 'new institutionalism' approach (Powell and DiMaggio 1991) with some emphasis on the notion of social embeddedness (Granovetter 1992; Moran 1999:10–12). The three parts will be integrated through a Foucauldian-tinted lens and reference to actor network theory.

Welfare state regimes and health care systems

In his ground-breaking book *The Three Worlds of Welfare Capitalism* (1990), Esping-Andersen he presents us with a description, some history and an analysis of the variants of the welfare state in Europe and North America. The basic assumption is that states have found it necessary or desirable for social stability (or solidarity) to circumvent the market and to make available social and health services directly to their population, a process referred to as 'de-commodification'. The form this de-commodification takes systematically varies according to a three-fold typology of welfare state regimes: Liberal; Conservative Corporatist; Social Democratic. This was derived from the analysis of large and impressive data sets collected over several years by Esping-Andersen (ibid.:ix–x). Despite the methodological strengths of the study, however, it does suffer from a particular weakness, and that is he overemphasises the ideal typification of USA, Germany and Sweden (Bagguley 1994:78–9) thereby underplaying or ignoring important variations and complexities within and between the regimes. Moreover, his approach tends to pay insufficient attention to the supporting pillars to the regimes, which, in addition to the state, include the market, community and family (Goodin and Rein 2001), a point that has particular relevance to any discussion of health care systems.

First, let us examine the question of the ideal typification: the Liberal model based on modest, means-tested provision for a low-income clientele and, in health care, Medicare and Medicaid services for the poor and elderly; in short, the US approach. It is, however, an appellation also extended to the UK although the regime is much more of a hybrid, with co-existing sedimentary elements of social democratic forces that played an important role in the establishment of the National Health Service (NHS). Esping-Andersen (1990:166–67) suggests that this very success created institutional barriers to the further growth of social democracy because it was impossible to forge any alliance between organised labour (trade unions) and the welfare state. In some ways this is insightful for it does account for the modest achievements (and underresourcing) of the NHS in the UK. This does not mean, however, that the UK welfare state regime is wholly a liberal archetype.

The second type, Conservative Corporatist refers to those continental European countries who, in the area of health care services, opted for a hypothecated system of funding based on 'sickness funds' (that is, mutual insurance associations commonly based on occupation). Particularly important in the development of this model was Bismarck, the German Chancellor of the nineteenth century. In contra-distinction to both the Liberal and Social Democratic models, the corporatist version was a conservative response to the threats of Marxism and socialism. The organisation of, for example, the sickness funds emphasised status distinctions based on occupation at the same time as it provided support. The conservativeness of these corporate regimes need not be overemphasised for all of them have had to adapt to social democratic and socialist governments and programmes, and the corporatist system has had to adapt and change to reflect this. Nevertheless there remains an underlying commitment to social solidarity historically based on the church and family ('subsidiarity') over liberal concerns for market efficiency or social democratic ones for equality.

Perhaps the closest match between ideal type and actuality is the third variety, the Social Democratic found in Scandinavia. Here the purpose of the welfare state is to promote social equality and services of the highest standard (ibid.: 27) and there is little substantial variation between Sweden and the other Scandinavian countries as compared to the corporate varieties in Continental Europe. The approach is neither minimalist, as in the case of the liberal regimes, nor has it the conservative intent of protecting the status quo and maintaining status differentials. The aims were rooted in working-class aspirations and are sustained by those of the new middle classes.

There is one particular group of countries that Esping-Andersen's ideal typology fails to deal with satisfactorily and that is the Southern European countries (Italy, Greece, Portugal and Spain). All these public sector health systems are based on a national health system model ostensibly similar too but distinctively different from the NHS of the UK. The same ambivalence between socialist (or social democratic) aspiration, cost-efficiency and class settlement also underpins Southern European states' adoption of a national health system model as was true of the UK. What is different, however, is that the historical and political legacies are corporate and autocratic, not liberal and conservative. Consequently, the cultural expectations of the citizens and the professions may well be more akin to the 'state-corporatist' of Germany or France than that of the UK. Katrougalos (1996:43), for instance, suggests that the southern welfare states are 'merely underdeveloped species of the continental [that is corporatist] model'. There is much to commend this view, particularly if one views the apparently underdeveloped sense of social solidarity as merely an aspect of late development. Another observer, Ferrera (1996), commenting on this point stated: [S]ome voices...lament...southern Europe...is...doomed to remain a second-rate periphery. Others argue...[that European] integration...represents a good chance for...finally aligning the still under-developed Mediterranean littoral with the more civilised [*sic*] European inland' (p. 34). On the other hand, the limited success that these states have had incorporating family loyalties and clientelism into a system of subsidiarity may be deeply embedded in the social and political fabric. Rather than the community and family providing the supporting pillars to the regimes (Goodin and Rein 2001) they operates as alternatives to it.

There is yet another group that might be thought of as late developers, although for very different reasons, and these are the East European countries, all of whom were state socialist (that is, communist) until the late 1980s and early 1990s. While not included in Esping-Andersen's

(1990) original analysis they are discussed by Standing (1996). Here too economic factors have played a large part in limiting these states' capacity to provide a comprehensive system of welfare and health services in recent times. Unlike the Southern European countries, however, these states have shown a greater willingness – at least initially – to adopt the shock therapy of market liberalisation solutions (Standing 1996:230–1). My conclusion is that while Esping-Andersen's ideal type triptych of Liberal, Corporate and Social Democratic regimes provides a helpful but limited typology, it is more useful, for example, than the Bismarck versus Beveridge distinction, which fails even to differentiate between the UK hybrid and the Scandinavian regimes and their health care systems. The welfare state regimes model does have the merit of providing a good basis for differentiating between the range of health care systems across Europe and their responses to any global trends in public management. However, for my purposes it is useful to extend the typology from three ideal types to five descriptive categories derived from the welfare state regimes:

1 continental Corporate (Germany, France and Benelux countries)
2 Social Democratic (Scandinavia)
3 Neo-liberal hybrid (UK)
4 Southern European (Italy, Greece, Spain and Portugal)
5 Eastern 'transitional' societies (for example, Poland, Hungary, Czech Republic).

These can be represented diagrammatically (see Figure 2.1). The diagram places Social Democratic and Corporatist regimes at opposite ends of the horizontal axis, representing the two 'pure' types of approaches to health care funding and provision in Europe. The vertical axis discriminates between the more 'hybridised' types of regimes – 'Neo-liberal', 'Southern European' and 'transitional'. The case study chapters (3–6) are organised so that each pairing of countries ensures a comparison between regimes.

The medical and nursing professions

The distinctions between welfare state regimes also provide the basis for the analysis of European nursing and medical professions. I start with the nursing profession and the issue of gender because it is in part a critical discussion Esping-Andersen's work. Also, in the analysis of nursing and professionalism, issues around variations in the social and cultural

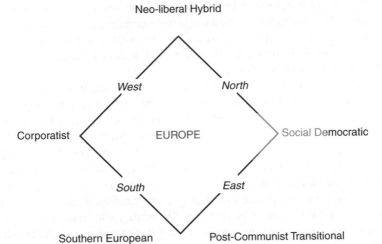

Figure 2.1 European welfare state regimes and health care systems

embeddedness of health care can be clearly identified. This in turn is a useful precursor to the comparative analysis of the medical profession and the interrelations between the two health professions.

Nursing, professionalisation and gender

The issue of gender and professionalisation of nursing, at least in the English language literature, has been dominated by North American, Australasian and UK debates. The predicament of nurses in Continental Europe, despite commonalities, is rather different. This partly reflects a different history and organisation of professions across much of Europe within which nursing has had great difficulty in translating professional aspirations into any practical reality, for nurses are locked into a well-established, institutionalised adjunct role to the doctors even more than nurses within Anglo-Saxon countries. But that is not the only reason. Nurse education and training across continental Europe is often perceived as being of lower status relative to other kinds of professional and technical work, and the root of that prejudice lies elsewhere. Burrage, Jarausch and Siegrist (1990), in their proposal for an actor-based framework for the study of the professions, argue that we should look at the occupations' relations with four sets of actors: the practising professionals, their clients, the state and the universities. They also suggest, following Abbott (1988), that other professions might also be included.

This is a helpful approach but inadequate for addressing the issue of gender and professionalism, and more so in certain parts of Europe than others. While gender relations are reproduced within the workplace and related institutions they also lie embedded within a broader network of family and social relations.

In this section of the chapter I will review the feminists' critique of Esping-Andersen's (1990) welfare state regimes model and in the process bring into the discussion consideration of the social institutions and principles that are central to the understanding of, and variations between, the different welfare state regimes. These include, importantly, subsidiarity, familialism and clientelism. First, however, I will revisit some of the North American and UK literature on the nursing professionalisation project before extending to the broader European dimension. The rationale here is that the US and, to a lesser extent, UK accounts are often taken to represent the future for professional nursing without taken into account significant cultural and social difference.

The relations between nursing and medicine within the division of labour has come to reflect a situation that, despite professional aspirations early in their modern development, has meant nursing remaining at risk of subordination to medicine (Abbott 1988:71–3). This raises the provocative question whether nursing is really a profession at all? In the North American literature nursing was often assumed to be a semi-profession. The conclusion from a classic text from this genre stated:

> Hospital nurses...point...out that the heart of being a professional nurse is a commitment to personal care of patients, not a commitment to abstract systems of knowledge. From this point of view, the traditional hospital arrangement that makes the nurse subservient to physicians but autonomous in regard to nurturent care is a viable system. (Katz 1969:76)

Hence the notion of 'semi-' professional, as the occupation can only ever be partly autonomous. This observation continues to have resonance for nurses across Europe and the fact that the quote comes from thirty years ago is a telling one, as is Katz's accompanying comment:

> The new professional aspirations [of nurses] with their focus on the nurse as a scientific colleague of the physician hold the promise of making personalized care increasingly sophisticated. But hospitals will have to develop adequate arrangements for translating the new sophistication of nurses into workable organizational patterns. (ibid.)

Sociological concepts sometimes hurt peoples' feelings and this seems to have been the case with 'semi-professions', but it is also the case that it has serious theoretical weaknesses. The term itself is imprecise and in any case suffers from the tautological weaknesses of the functionalist framework within which it is located (see Johnson 1972). By the 1980s, the distinction (between 'semi' and 'full' professions) had been replaced by the more neutral terms of 'autonomous' and 'heteronomous' professions. This drew upon the Weberian distinction between an autonomous profession whose members' control over their work and organisation was independent of any state or other bureaucratic mediation, and the heteronomous where they did not (Larson 1977). Social workers and teachers, for instance, rely on the state to provide them with clients. Nurses are similar, except that their work has and is often mediated by another profession – the autonomous doctors. Here Abbott's (1988: 87–91; 96) concept of jurisdiction is useful. The term means a profession's control over its work and its interdependence, influence and possible dominance over other professions. This approach emphasises the dynamic processes by which professions are socially constructed in competition with other occupations and professions. The medical profession has been particularly successful in controlling and dominating the health care division of labour and in the process circumscribing the nurses' professionalisation project. Thus, according to this interpretation nursing would only 'professionalise' fully when it could carve out significant areas of specialised work which – faced with the powerful jurisdiction of the medical profession – has proven extremely difficult. The issue that was overlooked in this account of the 'semi' and heterogenous professions and jurisdictions is that of gender. Both social work and teaching have high female membership but neither can match that of nursing where the figure is generally well over 90 per cent (see individual chapters). The public perception of nursing is that it is women's work (for example, Davies 1995:2), and Witz (1992:43–53) has drawn on the concept of 'occupational closure' to account for the gender dynamics of the professionalisation project of UK nurses and midwives. This, she argues, was an attempt at 'occupational imperialism' (Larkin 1983) pursued from a position of strategic weakness, a project intended to both resist the domination of the medics (that is, doctors determining nursing work) and create an autonomous work domain (ibid.:50). The problem, however, for such a project, as Witz makes clear, is that professionalisation is a masculine project within patriarchal societies (Hearn 1982). It is important, however, not to elide the distinctions between women/men and our historically and culturally constructed femininities/masculinities (for example, Butler, 1990; Davies 1996:663; Brunni and Gheradi 2002:177–9). It is not the consequence that, historically, men have, more or less, exclusively staffed the professions. Instead, the argument is that the professions reproduce patriarchal structures and relations within society. The work and organisational relations between nursing and medicine have mirrored these broader structures to the disadvantage of nursing, although this is not to suggest this will always be the case.

The erosion of the certainties of the welfare state, coupled with the introduction of neo-liberal and managerialist agendas has begun to change the discourse on the professions across society and business (Dent and Whitehead 2002). Even the classic autonomous and dominant professions of medicine and law have been subjected to increasing external regulation and control. The professional autonomy of hospitals doctors, for instance, is no longer a sufficient basis for medical dominance within hospitals. The emergence of post-bureaucratic, flexible and networked organisations, coupled with an emphasis on the notion of consumerism and the associated spread of the logic of the market, has undermined our pre-existing assumptions concerning professionalism and expert labour (Hanlon 1998; Fournier 1999, 2000:77–8). These broader changes affecting expert labour may well be advantageous to the organised nursing professions across Europe. The 'new' professionalism may not necessarily be based on the binary gendered thinking that underpins pre-existing notions of the professions (Davies 1996:673) for neither 'markets' nor 'managerialism' are premised on such distinctions. However, it is important not to be sanguine; this 'new' professionalism may not break the domination of masculine values and performativity (Whitehead 2002:134–7).

Nursing, gender and welfare state regimes

It is the question of gendered relations within the different European countries, in particular in relation to welfare state regimes and health care systems, that I now turn. Esping-Andersen's (1990) analysis, based as it is on de-commodification (p. 47), initially attracted critical reviews from feminist analysts (for example, Lewis 1992; O'Connor 1993, 1996; Orloff 1993; Sainsbury 1994). This was on the grounds that, as O'Connor (1993) in particular, pointed out: 'before de-commodification becomes an issue for individuals a crucial first step is access to the labour market. The de-commodification concept does not take into account the fact that not all demographic groups are equally commodified and that this may be a source of inequality' (p. 512).

Women in particular are most likely to be 'constrained by caring responsibilities' from fully entering the labour market unless there a range of child care and 'family-friendly' policies in place. Hence, all welfare state regimes are gendered to a greater or lesser extent, and all are to some degree 'male-breadwinner' (that is, patriarchal) states (Lewis 1992). For working women, including nurses, therefore, the issue of gender is not only matter of patriarchy operating within the workplace. It extends beyond this and, in the case of nurses, influences the relations between themselves and patients as well as the state in addition to those between themselves and doctors.

In Figure 2.2, based on Trifiletti's (1999:54) typology, the dimensions of gender and de-commodification are placed together on the x and y axes to create four logical cells for four, not three, welfare state regimes. Gender discrimination as identified by Lewis (1989:595) is placed on the horizontal axis and Esping-Andersen's de-commodification distinction on the vertical axis. This fourth cell provides the logical space for Southern European welfare state regimes as well as, possibly, the transitional regimes of Eastern Europe. The gender distinction is between those welfare state regimes that view women as 'wives and mothers' and those where women are treated primarily as 'workers'.

The Breadwinner regimes of the corporatist states assume women are not principally engaged in the labour market but concerned more with family matters (that is, social reproduction). Hence health and social

	State considers women as wives and mothers	State considers women as workers
State protects from market	**BREADWINNER** (Corporatist)	**UNIVERSALIST** (Social Democratic)
	Maximum gender discrimination	Minimum gender discrimination
State does not protect from market	**CLIENTELISTIC** (Southern European or Transitional)	**MINIMALIST** (Liberal)

Figure 2.2 A typology of welfare state regimes
Source: [Trifiletti 1999:54 *slightly modified*]

entitlements are premised on the occupation of the male breadwinner. The underlying ideology is heavily imbued with the principle of subsidiarity 'the state will only interfere when the family's capacity to service its members is exhausted' (Esping-Andersen 1990:27). Historically, this is the policy of the (Catholic) Church, although in its de-sanctified form it translates as the state supports the family to help itself. The Universalist regime (Social Democratic), by contrast, is one that treats women principally as workers. The rationale of the regime is to provide social and health services that ensure adequate support for child care, maternity/paternity leave, care of the elderly and so on in order that women (along with men) may remain active in the labour market. The Liberal (minimalist) regime is one that accepts women are workers but does little to protect them from the labour market. It more or less ignores their family roles, expecting them instead to make their own care arrangements. Only in the case of poverty will the system deliver any support. Within Europe the UK is the key exponent of this approach; it shares some similarities with the Southern European countries but there are some crucial differences. The Mediterranean countries have an ambiguous approach to female employment. On the one hand, the public view is one of accepting that women are workers but privately (that is, domestically) assuming men should be the breadwinners. The outcome is that there is little support for childcare, care of elderly people and not much protection within the labour market. Despite some similarities, there is a significant difference between the Mediterranean and Transitional regimes. In the case of the Southern European (Mediterranean) countries this results from the state treating women (along with men) principally on the basis of their family roles and, historically, seeing little reason to provide protection for them if they enter the labour market (Trifiletti 1999:54). In the case of the Transitional countries of Eastern Europe the state formally recognise women as workers but, unlike the Universalist regimes, has been unable to provide much protection from the market. There is some evidence however that these states may be moving more towards more of a Breadwinner model of Western Europe, and this is reflected in more recent social and health policies (see Chapter 6). To elaborate this argument, the Southern European (Mediterranean) regimes are the consequence of late – capitalist – development (Ferrera 1996; Katrougalas 1996) and, while a parallel argument may be made in relation to post-communist Eastern Europe, the nature of their lateness is a little different for they followed another path, one that took them through nearly half a century of state socialist rule. There is another dimension not captured in the diagram but which may discriminate between Southern and Eastern Europe. This is the issue of clientelism that is differentially distributed across these groups of countries. Clientelism might be viewed as a particular variant of subsidiarity in that it consists of a local network of loyalty and obligations but is not formalised or legitimated in anything like the same way as subsidiarity. It has a long history in most Mediterranean countries – Greece, Italy, Spain and Portugal – where it has underpinned, and continues in varying degrees to underpin, political, social and family life. A version also exists in all Eastern European countries although it would appear to be a more pragmatic variety that emerged under the communist regimes and for that reason may possibly be less deeply embedded within the social fabric of these societies.

Subsidiarity, familialism and clientelism – and social embeddedness

It is the issues of subsidiarity, clientelism plus a third category, familialism, that are crucial to our understanding of gender and welfare state regimes. They relate to the socially embedded values attributed to paid care (including nursing). Unlike the Universalistic and Liberal regimes, nursing within the Breadwinner and Southern European types commonly enjoys low status and pay rates, even where the occupation has a strong sense of professional identity. To explain the reason why this should be so it is necessary first to examine these categories of subsidiarity, familialism and clientelism in more detail.

Subsidiarity.   was originally the principle that the state should only intervene when the family is unable to provide for itself (Esping-Andersen, 1990:61). The concept is central to the Corporatist regimes, which has meant that these states have tended not to provide those services that enable mothers (and other caregivers) to readily enter the labour market (Orloff 1993:312). The principal in relation to the family and its relations with the state is not restricted to the Catholic Church, for the Protestant churches in Germany and The Netherlands are also strongly supportive of the principle. Subsidiarity has also become a much broader political and social principle that has come to mean the state should not intervene if other social collectivities can provide the service. In German health care, for instance, church 'not-for-profit' hospitals have the legal right to operate alongside public hospitals and receive public funding.

Familialism.   refers to the centrality of the (patriarchal) extended family network and its obligations within the social and political system.[1] This is the institutional reciprocal of subsidiarity but also exists independently of it, for it also correlates strongly with clientelism.

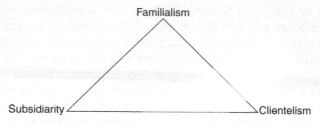

Figure 2.3 Subsidiarity, familialism and clientelism

Clientelism. is that form of patronage that 'has been extraordinarily influential in taming the brutal world of commodification' (Esping-Andersen 1990:139). In one form it is where an employer provides, for example, health facilities and housing for employees and education for their children. It can take on a corrupt form too, as where, for example, health professionals expect to be bribed for the work they do (see Chapter 6). It is perhaps best known in connection with Southern Italy (for example, Putnam 1993) and can be extended to the post-communist transitional countries of Eastern Europe.

These three categories or practices and their interconnections are represented in Figure 2.3, for while familialism remains a constant, subsidiarity and clientelism are alternatives for each other: subsidiarity is a principle that can only apply if the state is well organised and with sufficient power to make that choice. Thus, for example, within the established corporatist regimes one finds a strong commitment to the principle, although France – with its *étatiste* tradition – is an exception. In the cases of Greece and Poland (Chapter 6) the state does not enjoy the ascendancy it does in France. In these cases, and other Southern and Eastern European countries too, clientelism is not so much a component of subsidiarity but an alternative to it. The reason for this is that within a Breadwinner regime the three corners of the triangle are integrally configured and buttress each other, whereas within the Mediterranean and Transitional regimes the state lacks the resources to legislate for subsidiarity. In this case the welfare state regime is constantly subject to the centrifugal force of special interests of clientelism and familialism. The problem, according to Ferrera (1996:125) is the 'double deficit of "stateness"'. While Ferrera developed the notion to explain problems within the Italian health care system, it is also more generally applicable. First, the central state is unable to adequately control welfare institutions. The regional authorities or other countervailing forces prove to be too powerful. Second, the state is unable to prevent public institutions being vulnerable to partisan pressure and manipulation. In this case the welfare state regime is constantly subject to the centrifugal force of special interests of clientelism and familialism.

Implications for nursing

Nursing is universally an occupation that is gendered female yet the implications of this are not the same across Europe. In very broad terms, within the Breadwinner and Southern European regimes their stronger familial and clientelist values have meant that nursing generally has been viewed as being of lower status than in the Universalist and Liberal regimes, for following reason. Familial values mean that the family has the prime responsibility to care for its members who are sick, while nurses tend to be viewed as analogous to domestic servants or in some cases there are religious connotations with nurses being equated with nuns, that is dedicated to service and humility. Consequently, the nursing role is not viewed by the general public as a professional one but as one that can be carried out by women of with minimal qualifications. The differences with the Universalist and Liberal regimes should not be overstated, for here too entry into nursing does not require the level of educational attainment of other professions, and the oral traditions and practical nature of nursing are a recognised component of the nursing identity. At the same time, however, patients and their families are not threatened by an loss of face if they are cared for in hospitals by nurses with family inputs limited to regular visits and emotional support.

This analysis of European nursing has so far treated the profession within each country as an undifferentiated one. This fails to take account of the internal components of nursing and for that reason it will be useful to address the issue of segmentation.

Segmentation

Another aspect of the question 'is nursing "really" a profession or not?' relates to whether the activities of nursing comprise one occupation or contain elements of several which, if integrated in a certain way, could be seen as a profession, but generally this had not happened. It is useful here to draw on the well-established concept of 'segmentation'. Bucher and Strauss (1961) first introduced the concept of professional segmentation with reference to medicine and defined a profession as a 'loose amalgamation of segments that are in movement'. Thus in medicine the specialties are the 'segments' and these are in dynamic relation with each other and with other occupations as well as their clientele. But they are all effectively committed to the organised profession of medicine. This has not proven to be the case with nursing. In the UK context Carpenter (1977) distinguished three main segments within nursing: 'new managers', 'new professionals' and 'rank and file'. The term 'new' is anachronistic now for it refers to developments in the 1960s and 1970s when nurse management was introduced into the UK NHS and a relatively small group of clinical nurse specialists also emerged almost as a 'counter-culture' to this nurse managerialism. This development followed the lead of the US nursing profession. The 'rank and file', by contrast, apparently enjoyed the reflected status of working for and alongside doctors. Melia (1987) later added the 'academic professionalisers' to the mix. This group (segment) seeks to achieve autonomy for nursing based on the academic credibility of nursing theory and research. The problem for nursing is that often these groups are more like factions than segments and they have divided rather than integrated the occupation. It may be that what these segments reveal are the overlapping domains of nursing and care reflecting different ratios of indeterminancy/technicity (Jamous and Peloille 1970). Thus general rank and file nursing may well be vulnerable to rationalisation and nurses' work being delegated to less qualified personnel (for example, health care assistants) whereas the nurse specialists and academics are not. The indeterminancy of these groups (segments), however, may derive more from their academic and/or medical connections than directly from nursing. The managerialist segment may also comprise more managers than professionals, at least when working at the more senior levels. These segments are also to be found to a greater or lesser extent across Europe although the influence of US nursing practice appears to have been less immediate and direct than the case of nursing within the UK. There are, however, considerable differences between countries that are in part a consequence of the variations in the patterns of gender relations and identity within the wider society. Another dimension to this difference between regimes is the role of the doctors. Under the Liberal and Universalist regimes the development of various forms of advanced nursing (for example, nurse practitioners) carrying out clinical work that historically had been the domain of doctors is seen as acceptable and even desirable by the nursing profession, the doctors and the public. Within the Breadwinner and Southern European and Transitional regimes this is not the case and advanced clinical practice has little or no appeal. Nursing is about caring for patients – not treatment.

Nurse professionalisation projects

The main influences shaping the success or otherwise of nurse professionalisation within any particular country's health system will be the following:

- type of welfare state regime and the implications this has for gender
- number of doctors relative to population and their expectations of nurses
- the labour market
- nurse management within hospitals.

The issue of the relationship between welfare state regime and gender and the implications for nursing has already been discussed in some detail. This is also interconnected to the interesting fact that different European countries produce different numbers of doctors relative to their population and that it is among those countries with the greatest gender discrimination that the largest number of doctors are trained. Moreover, there would seem to be little evidence that medical schools would ever fail to fill their student places. Whereas in the case of nurses the opposite would appear to be the case: the more there are trained doctors the fewer nurses there are and the more difficult it is to attract recruits into nursing. Moreover, in those countries where there is an overproduction of doctors the more problems confront the organised nursing profession. The professional status of nurses, however, is not simply about medical jurisdiction (Abbott 1988) or doctors and nurse numbers; the labour market is also a critical factor. Nursing tends to provide relatively secure but not highly paid employment as a consequence, expanding or buoyant economies have problems recruiting nurses while stagnant economies or those in crisis tend not to (for example, see the comparison between northern and southern Italy). This exogenous factor can to some extent be mitigated if nursing has been able to gain senior management positions within the hospital hierarchy (as well as within the broader health service bureaucracy) in order to ensure the case for nursing is fully taken into account in strategic decision making. It will be these factors that will be examined in relation to nursing and by this means linked into the analysis of medical work and hospital organisation across Europe.

The medical profession, autonomy and the labour process

The position of doctors across Europe has been rather different from that of nurses. In part this has been a consequence of the profession being gendered male, which has also underpinned the dominant role of the profession within the health care division of labour and in relations with the state (for example, Abbott 1988:67).

Professional autonomy and medical work

During the period following 1945 when the Welfare State became part of the bedrock of European democracies, the state(s) became dependent on the medical profession as the arbiter of the quality and content of health care delivery. There were and are subtle variations between the states but broadly the following holds for them all. In medicine the organised profession comprises associations, colleges, chambers and so on, and while there are variations between countries, broadly speaking there will be a body that oversees the conduct and ethical practice of the membership and it is this organisation with which the government will rely on in matters relating to medical and health policy as well as medical education and training. Another constituency here, however, is that of the universities (for example, Abbott 1988:195–211; Burrage, Jarausch and Siegrist 1990:207) and in the corporate countries of continental Europe and southern Europe they can have a significant influence on the numbers of medical students (*numerus clausus*) as well as inhibiting the degree to which practical clinical medicine impinges on the curriculum. More generally, the organised medical profession in several European countries is closely integrated with the state (for example, *l'Ordre de Médecins* in France and its equivalent in Italy and Greece) whereas in others they are constitutionally independent (for example, Germany and The Netherlands). Scandinavia is different again and in the case of Sweden, for example, the medical profession has long been closely integrated with the state. In the case of UK, however, the relationship between the profession and state has long been ambivalent. Historically this has been a consequence of the organised profession having established its legal autonomy by the mid nineteenth century and was well established before the rise of the Welfare State in the twentieth. Instead, the profession was able to better exploit the market for medical services provided by the growing numbers of urban middle classes (Johnson 1972:52). Medical doctors in other European countries also benefited from the growth of the middle classes in the same period but their professional autonomy was more constrained by state regulation and the universities (Abbott 1988:58–162; Siegrist 1990; Macdonald 1995:98). This did not prohibit German and Dutch medical professions, for example, successfully establishing their variant of medical dominance on their countries, health care systems, but doctors in France and Italy, by contrast, were rather less successful (see Chapters 3, 4 and 5). Depending on this state–professional relationship were the other components of an organised profession, the scholarly associations and unions playing varying roles, sometime as independent forum or voice that the official body cannot provide (for example, Italy and Greece), in other places the distinction between professional and union matters are not clearly differentiated (for example, Sweden).

Professional autonomy equates to the legal standing of the organised medical profession which provides doctors with a monopoly over medical and surgical work. In return the profession is required to ensure it is properly self-regulated, which traditionally is a function carried out by the *l'Ordre de Médecins* in France, the General Medical Council in the UK and equivalent bodies in the other European countries. This institutional arrangement provides the umbrella for medical autonomy, a rather imprecise term that blurs the distinction between formal autonomy and actual medical practice, which directly relates to the concepts of 'de-coupling' (Meyer and Rowan 1991) and 'loose coupling' (Weick 1976) (see below). The rationale for this relative autonomy existing between formal regulation and actual practice is the complexity of certain aspects of medical work even if these are at times overstated or ambiguous (Jamous and Peloille 1970; Freidson 1994:87) and over recent years has become increasingly subject to budgetary limitations. Doctors are expected to make sound decisions (clinical judgements) drawing on their medical education, socialisation and experience, but since medicine is not a precise science there is room to argue over which is the most cost-effective as well as efficacious therapy. At the individual level there is the clinical autonomy of doctor, here the physician's discretion is being constrained by the introduction of new generations of quality assurance and clinical governance systems across many European countries including, in particular, clinical guidelines and evidence-based medicine. Clinical guidelines have their roots in medical audit, which in turn originated in the USA from a desire on part of US doctors to improve medical care, protect themselves from litigation and/or deal with the pressures of accreditation. This all led to the development of, first, criteria audits and subsequently medical protocols (or clinical guidelines a term perceived as advice rather than a demand to the profession). These were the standard procedures laid down by senior medics for their medical staff to follow. This summary indicates that 'medical protocols' (that is, clinical guidelines) may have been developed, paradoxically, not to erode medical autonomy but to protect it. Ellwood (1988), in an influential article, has presented a case to the medical profession in support of clinical guidelines. He argued for the introduction of a new system of 'outcomes management' (ibid.:1551) based on four techniques:

1   established standards and guidelines
2   systematic measurement of clinical outcomes
3   pooling of this data
4   data to be analysed and disseminated.

The process would become a 'clinical trial machine' (ibid.:1552) of the kind advocated by Cochrane (1972) and now known as evidence-based medicine (Eddy 1990a, 1990b; Sackett *et al*. 1996). The system was not to be seen as part of a management-led quality control system such as total quality management (TQM). Ellwood was not blind to some of the dangers (for the profession) of his proposals and acknowledged that it might be seen as 'cookbook medicine' (ibid.:1553) of the McDonaldized type (Ritzer 1996) – 'a bureaucrats paradise' (Ellwood 1988:1553). But clinical guidelines were not only the initiative of writers and activists from within the medical profession. Another important motivation for the adoption of quality assurance practices within European medicine was the World Health Organisation's 'Targets for Health for All by the Year 2000' (WHO 1985). This included the statement, 'By 1990, all member states should have built effective mechanisms for ensuring the quality of patient care within their health care systems' (ibid.116, quoted in Jost 1990:7). The WHO project appears all 'motherhood and apple pie' but there were complicating and even contradictory issues of efficiency and equity that needed to be taken into account. This issue is discussed within each of the case study chapters. Clinical guidelines and related practices impinge directly on the clinical freedom of individual doctors and this development suggests a fundamental change has occurred in the nature of medical dominance and clinical autonomy. Many European doctors now appear able – although not necessarily willing – to accept that their work will be routinely subject to external scrutiny of some kind. These changes to medical and clinical autonomies also reflect a broader sea change in health policies across a range of countries. In the last decades of the twentieth century various European governments began to try out a variety of ways of delivering 'financially sustainable, socially equitable and, ultimately, politically successful health care reform' (Figueras, Saltman and Sakellarides 1998:1). As mentioned earlier, there was in the 1980s and 1990s the introduction of the quasi-market approach, which was particularly influential in The Netherlands, UK and Sweden. This early variant of New Public Management (NPM) has given way more to that of managed care based on the USA Health Maintenance Organisation model (Light 1997; Ranade 1998:6–7). This has had most impact within the UK but the Dunning Committee in The Netherlands also advocated a managed care solution to providing effective and efficient health care services (van der Grintern and Kasdorp 1999). More generally, however, governments across Europe have been keen to find ways of containing the growth of health care expenditures – a consequence, primarily, of developments in medical technologies (including drugs), demographic changes and peoples' expectations. Therefore, containing these costs will have one or more effect: restrict citizens' access to health care; impose constraints on what the doctors can prescribe; limit what the public sector (including sickness funds) will pay for. It has been these circumstances that have provided the backdrop to concerns within the medical profession that the work of doctors has become increasingly rationalised and their autonomy curtailed. Such changes, it is believed by their advocates, will improve the efficiency and quality of the medical services. The question arises whether these changes reflect any kind of proletarianisation or deskilling of hospital doctors. Has their pre-existing dominance within the health care division of labour and its organisation been sufficiently eroded by quasi-market forces that they are now merely a group of skilled employees? To explore this possibility it is useful to interrogate labour process theory (Braverman 1974) and its relevance (or otherwise) to public sector organisations.

Labour process theory and the medical profession

Public sector services, particularly health, have played an important legitimising role within all capitalist societies (Habermas 1976; Offe 1984) and the work of the professionals and managers within it has played an important 'stabilising (or legitimating) function' in this process (Exworthy and Halford 1999:9). These services have been premised on the production of use values, 'however distorted' some may consider these to be (Thompson 1990:110), and not exchange values, more commonly associated with the market. In Esping-Andersen's (1990) argument they are de-commodified. However, this premis has been seriously challenged over recent years by neo-liberal ideology and the introduction of quasi-market principles. While the force of the ideology may well have abated, the impact on health care organisations should not be underestimated. Nevertheless, it would be incorrect to equate the public management reforms of this period as representing simply an abandonment of the public sector's legitimising role in favour of market economics. The health services, as the key example, are defined primarily by political rather than economic criteria even when operating under regulated market conditions. It is the state, not the market, that ultimately makes the decisions on resourcing issues even if priorities under a 'control and command' bureaucracy are very different from those applying under conditions of a quasi-market or managed care.

It is within the public sector environment that we find the professions have developed a particularly distinct role, for without the market to dictate priorities it has been the professions, to a greater or lesser extent, that have been responsible for defining them. The relationship between state and the professions appears to parallel that of *responsible autonomy* (Friedman 1977:78), not least because professionally organised occupational groups are differentiated from other groups because of their central role within the division of labour. There is, nevertheless, a crucial difference between responsible and professional autonomies (Dent 1993): responsible autonomy is the outcome of deliberate management strategies whereas professional autonomy is not. The latter reflects more the success of the profession's own strategy to gain control over the work and who is qualified to do it. There are parallels here with the concept of 'jurisdiction' (Abbott 1988) except that Abbott emphasises much more the relations between professional/occupational groups rather than with management. The distinction between a state-defined responsible autonomy and an independent professional status might be said to be that which lies between organisational and institutional control. Organisational control refers to the rules imposed by management in order to control costs and/or quality. Institutional control, by contrast, refers to the ability of an organized profession to define its members' autonomy within the workplace. It is important to note, however, that the distinction between organisational and institutional control is, in reality, far from clear-cut. Both types of control can and do co-exist uneasily together and the autonomy of doctors is something that is constantly being renegotiated. An example of this was the introduction of NPM in several countries across Europe, a process that can be viewed as being partly motivated by a desire to exert greater organisational control over doctors in order to control the costs and quality of treatment. One important outcome has been a much clearer separation between *allocative* and *operational* decisions within the health services. Doctors within the UK, for instance, are no longer able to commit additional resources as an outcome of their clinical decisions alone but have to work within predetermined budgets (Flynn 1992:79–103) and similar changes are occurring elsewhere in Europe. Doctors retain their control over their work (operational decisions), but allocative decisions are now much more clearly the preserve of management *qua* management. Even so, the dividing line between doctoring and managing at the local level (for example, hospital) is not a clear-cut one and members of the medical profession pursue careers as senior hospital managers in many parts of Europe. These changes do not, however, constitute any 'proletarianisation' of doctors, for, as McKinlay and Arches (1985:161) explained several years ago, they still retain their 'control over certain prerogatives relating to the location, content and essentiality of [their] task activities' (quoted in Elston 1991:63) even if they perceive themselves as suffering a loss of occupational status as Larson (1980), Derber (1982) and Derber, Schwartz, and Magrass 1990:122–5) have also argued some time ago. Nevertheless, in many parts of Europe doctors are coming under increasing organisational controls dictated by the state, and while this has not been at the expense of the doctors' dominant position within the health care division of labour it has meant that they have had to accept the state exercising greater suzerain power than was previously the case.

A similar argument has been popularised by Ritzer (1996), although one that draws more on Weber than Marx and goes under the rubric of the 'McDonaldisation'. The pressures to control costs and increase efficiency, so the argument runs, has led to a McDonaldisation of health care provision. There are, according to Ritzer (1996), four basic dimensions at the heart of the McDonald's model (pp. 9–11). First, *efficiency*, based on Taylorist and Fordist principles of work organization. Second, a service that can be *quantified* and *calculated* both in terms of how the tasks are performed and in the price and quality of the product. Third, *predictability*, so that no matter in which McDonald's restaurant you eat you always eat exactly the same food. Finally, *control* through replacing human skills and knowledge with technology. This system of control, however, is not exercised through any monolithic corporate or state hierarchy but via a tightly controlled franchising arrangement. There is a prima facie case that organisational reforms in health care have had a McDonaldising impact but important differences become apparent on closer examination. First, as with chefs working in cordon bleu restaurants, general hospitals continue to remain dependent upon the medical expertise and autonomy of the doctors. This limits the extent to which standardised routines (protocols) and new technologies can routinise the work. Second, measurement and assessment of the quality of service is not limited to the patients' (consumers') or managers' evaluations. Medical staffs, unlike those working at a McDonald's restaurant, have a claim to an expertise that only they can judge. Third, local management and professional staff have greater influence on the organization of hospitals than is the case with McDonald's restaurants. All of these elements limit the impact of NPM reforms and provide hospital doctors with a new repertoire of opportunities to take on an active and possibly leading role in the organisation and control of health care.

Another development discernible within labour process analysis has been a trend towards a Foucauldian informed analysis adopted originally perhaps as ready-made response to the widespread implementation of Just In Time (JIT) systems within manufacturing (for example, Sewell and Wilkinson 1992:271–89), a development paralleling the nineteenth-century panopticon (Foucault 1979a). The appropriateness here is reasonably obvious for 'discipline and punish' offers another way of looking at responsible autonomy but, unlike conventional labour process, conceptualising power relations not manifested as class struggle but as a web of complex relations that have given rise to a whole range of disciplinary mechanisms, surveillance techniques and power-knowledge strategies (Foucault 1981). This extends the analytical leverage of labour process theory, although it is true that such an innovation brings with it agnosticism, which is not strictly compatible with the emancipatory ideal of labour process theory (Thompson 1990). While not offering any universal truths, however, the theory is not incompatible with a delimited pragmatism.

Governmentality and the institutionalisation of expertise

One means of unravelling the relationship between the professions and public management reforms is to consider Foucault's discourse on governmentality, which broadly concerns the ensemble of institutions that ensure, more or less, the continuing reproduction of the self-regulating citizen-subject (Johnson 1995:12). It is in part another way of accounting for the legimating role of the health services (cf. Habermas 1976; Offe 1984) for it accounts for the mechanisms by which governments govern in line with 'the personal and collective conduct of subjects' (Johnson 1995:12) and this includes crucially the role of the professions. This contrasts with Durkheim's notion of the professions as the *corp-intermediaires* between 'laissez-faire individualism and state collectivism' (Johnson 1972:12) for it suggests that the professions are part of the process of governing in a wider sense. The form governmentality takes and the ways in which the institutionalised expertise of the professions operates will vary according to the particular history of the particular country. There are a number of insights to be gained from this approach. The professions, including both nursing and medicine, are to be seen as a 'key resource of governing in a liberal-democratic state' (Johnson 1995:23) which facilitates normalisation. Moreover, it draws attention to the possibility of changes in state–professions relations, for example as happened in the wake of the 'Thatcherite reforms in UK', to quote Johnson (1995:22): 'new jurisdictional claimants [were brought] into being [including]...appraisers, auditors and monitors of expert services'. This refers to the emergence of what Power (1994, 1997) has called the 'Audit Society' and one that impinges sharply on pre-existing notions of professional autonomy. This is a crucial component of the collection of managerial techniques that has come to be known as New Public Management, a phenomena that has been claimed to be more or less global in its impact and has had major implications for hospital medicine and nursing.

European hospitals, organisations and New Public Management

This section has two objectives. The first is to assess the relevance or otherwise of New Public Management (NPM) to account for the changes in hospital organisation and health care systems across Europe. The second is to construct a theoretical framework robust enough for the comparative analysis of changes in hospital organisation and medical and nursing work. This will draw on the earlier discussion on the sociology of the professions but will be primarily focused on the question of the usefulness or otherwise of the new institutionalism (Powell and DiMaggio 1991; Scott *et al.* 2000).

Public sector management reforms

Over the last twenty-five years or so, a portfolio of public management techniques has evolved and been applied, particularly but not solely within Anglo-Saxon countries. These techniques emerged initially in the form of increasing privatisation and marketisation of public services associated with the Reagonism and Thatcherism of the 1980s but have evolved as a sophisticated regulatory framework. This was initially rationalised by recourse to the 'new institutionalist economics' (Williamson 1975; Powell 1991), which provided the starting-point for a course that led to the abandonment of the Welfare State in favour of a far more minimalist approach to government justified in terms of 'the hollowing out of the state' which was better at 'steering than rowing' (Osborne and Gaebler 1992). A lean state is judged the more effective one, it is best to leave the delivery of services to other agencies and to rely, wherever possible, on competition and managerialism to provide the spur to efficiency and effectiveness. This is governance rather than government (see Pollitt and Bourckaert 2000:10–11). A principal commentator on this phenomena, Hood's (1991, 1995:95–7) has listed the components of what has come to be known as NPM as follows:

1   greater 'disaggregation' of public sector organisations into separately managed units
2   enhanced competition coupled with the use of private sector managerial techniques
3   greater user choice of service provider
4   emphasis on 'discipline and parsimony' in resource use
5   greater 'hands-on management'
6   adoption of measurable standards of performance
7   use of 'pre-set output measures'.

In more recent work Hood *et al.* (1999:191–3) have argued that NPM is becoming more concerned with surveillance (increased 'oversight') and regulation through mechanisms such as audit and the whole question of governance. Having identified its key characteristics and identified NPM as the major force for public management reforms, Hood (1995), however, resists strongly the Osborne and Gaebler view that NPM is the new global paradigm. For while there may be a diffusion of 'the same management buzzwords…on its own [this] is a trivial level of convergence' (ibid.:109). More important is the question whether the changes being described are sufficiently similar to be sensibly labelled New Public Management? Hood thinks not and for reasons similar to those suggested by Pollitt and Bouckaert (2000:60–1), namely that 'Anglo-Saxon' countries, including the UK and USA, appear to be 'more open to the "performance-driven", market-favouring ideas of NPM than others'. Among these 'others' are those European countries with a strong *Rechtsstaat* tradition within which the state has the central integrative role within society underpinned by a strong legal framework. It is a category that corresponds to the Conservative Corporatist regime identified by Esping-Andersen (1990) (discussed in detail earlier in this chapter) and of which France and Germany represent key examples. It is also the case that these two countries reflect the main contrast within regime type, with France representing the unitary and strongly centralised state (*étatiste*) and which has introduced some NPM-type reforms. Germany, on the other hand, is a federal state in which the individual states (*Länder*) have considerable constitutional powers that have been used to restrict the impact of any new managerialism (see Chapters 4 and 5).

NPM can be viewed as part of the armoury of neo-liberalism, arguably more an ideology (Clarke and Newman 1997) than a template for public sector management reforms, and it represents a challenge to the professions. This is especially so in relation to professional regulation, audit and the organisational governance (Power 1994, 1997; Jary 2002) and not least the medical and nursing professions. However, NPM has not fully permeated all the countries of Europe (more specifically the 'European Union' [EU]) although, as both Saltman (1997) and Pollitt (2001) have pointed out, there has been a growing convergence on the use of its terminology. Pollitt refers to NPM directly while Saltman does not, although he is discussing the same agenda; also, Pollitt's discussion covers management across all public sectors while Saltman is concerned specifically with health care systems. He argues that within health care the question of convergence or not is a complex one. He cites approvingly Wilsford's (1995) contention that the 'philosophy is convergent, but organizational principles and instruments are divergent' and suggests that there are three categories of analysis to be taken into account. These are the social, political and the technical (or 'mechanical'). The first, the social, embodies the core cultural characteristics of a society, which will reflect its history and dominant values and norms. The second, the political, is concerned with the national political goals and objectives and will change over time but, nevertheless, still reflect the underlying norms and values. The final category, the technical, includes crucially the following three elements: (1) scientific medicine; (2) institutional management; (3) provider payment mechanisms. This categorisation is a useful one for it alerts us to the dangers of assuming that because a certain vocabulary is used or a particular policy adopted, consistent with the principles of NPM, that is what is happening. Things may not be quite as they seem, perhaps there is in all this a substantial element of 'smoke and mirrors' or, to change the metaphor, 'myth and ceremony' (Meyer and Rowan 1991). At the social level, for example, Europeans (including the British) perceive health care primarily as a social good to be made collectively available, although there are substantial differences between countries how this is achieved. By contrast the USA continues to emphasise the role of the market and commercial aspects of health care provision and payment systems. At the political level there appears to be more convergence in the official policies but substantial differences in the willingness to implement them. Perhaps the most obvious case is that of The Netherlands, which was an early adopter of 'marketisation' (privatisation of sickness funds) but then retreated from this policy (see Chapter 3). A not dissimilar change of tack also occurred in the UK and Sweden – both early converts to these reforms. In the cases of the *Rechtsstaat* and Southern European countries the picture is more complex again (see Chapters 5 and 6). At the technical/mechanical level there does appear to be considerable convergence, particularly within medicine (around the principles of 'scientific medicine') despite cultural variations in its delivery, although, as Saltman asserts, 'considerably less convergence regarding organizational management within health systems' (op cit:451). There is also less convergence around nursing despite EU regulations on education and training. Saltman opposes 'convergence' with the notion of 'social embeddedness', drawing on Granovetter (1992) for inspiration and in the process sensitises us not only to the importance of cultural and social norms in explaining organisational and policy change but also to 'new institutionalism', if only because Granovetter's work has been incorporated within this broader body of theory. Pollitt's account (2001:945) is more direct in making this link, arguing that 'institutionalist theories enrich our model of the agent's cognition'. Moreover, in bringing 'agents back in' it is not at the expense of 'throwing structures and constraints out'. But one has to pick over new institutionalism carefully because, while it does provide a powerful theoretical framework for the comparative analysis of European health systems and organisations, it can also overemphasise the forces for convergence or, to use the new institutionalist terminology, 'isomorphism'.

New Institutionalism and health care organisations

Meyer and Rowan (1991) have been particularly influential in establishing New Institutionalism within organisational studies. DiMaggio and Powell (1991a:11) actually date its birth from the 1977 publication of their paper, 'Institutionalized organizations: formal structure as myth and ceremony' (reprinted in 1991). This set out much of the core components of the theory and, following Berger and Luckman (1967), with the emphasis on the socially constructed reality of organisations. New Institutionalism is not peculiar to organisational theory but it has impacted on the various social sciences, including policy analysis, in different ways, although the prioritising of values and norms is common to them all. Lowndes (1996:182) provides a useful 'baseline' definition of what is meant by 'institution' and 'institutions', which can be paraphrased as follows:

1 it is a middle-level (meso) concept – they are devised by humans yet shape their actions, imposing constraints and providing opportunities;
2 they are a mix of formal rules/ regulations and informal norms and customs;
3 they have legitimacy and stability through time.

In some ways the New Institutionalism has become the new 'systems theory', a putative integrative theory of the social sciences. In this it will probably fail for while the conceptual language may be universalised the processes and practices it draws on to describe and analyse may not be beyond a very general level. On another hand, the approach has some potential, particularly for cross-comparative studies.

New Institutionalism is so called to point up the continuity and differences from the older 'institutionalism' of Selznick (1949) and others (DiMaggio and Powell 1991a:12) who viewed organisations as reflecting their local environment. In contrast, the 'new' institutionalists take the view that organisations respond to a much wider 'organisational field'. To explain the import of this fundamental difference it is useful to quote directly from DiMaggio and Powell (1991a:13).

> Authors of the older works...describe organizations that are embedded in local communities, to which they are tied by the multiple loyalties of personnel and interorganizational treaties ('co-option') hammered out in face-to-face interaction. The new institutionalism focuses instead on non-local environments, either organizational sectors or *fields* roughly co-terminus with the boundaries of industries, professions, or national societies...*Environments*, in this view, are more subtle in their influence; rather than being co-opted by organizations, they penetrate the organization, creating the lenses through which actors view the world and the very categories of structure, action, and thought. (*emphases added*).

It is possibly simplistic, but nevertheless useful, to state that the two versions are not necessarily in conflict with one another. The values and cultures of particular organisations will be 'shaped' by their organisational fields more than the earlier institutionalists recognised. Similarly, the local environment may well be more influential than the new institutionalists are ready to acknowledge, especially when the discussion relates to cross-national comparisons. To be clear, I am equating local environment here not with a particular town or village community but with national and regional cultures (that is, socially embedded practices), for example 'Southern Italy' or 'Sweden'. It may be that in the cases of the oil industry, certain soft drinks (for example, Coca or Pepsi Cola) and fast-food restaurants (for example, McDonald'), local values and cultures have limited implications for the organisational field, but in the cases of many other organisations, particularly those operating within the public sector, this is not the case even though they will be heavily influenced by international and national agendas of governments and corporations (for example, pharmaceutical companies). Local – national or regional – values, norms and culture will often differ systematically from elsewhere. A good example of this is the case of NPM (as discussed earlier) and the degree to which it has and is being disseminated across the globe. Whilst it may appear to be ubiquitous, the form it takes and the priorities it is intended to address vary substantially between different countries and in different sectors within them (for example, education, police, local government, health care).

According to DiMaggio and Powell (1991b:67) the process of dissemination of new organisational and management practices is best understood in terms of 'isomorphism'. They provide a three-fold typology, *coercive, mimetic* and *normative* isomorphism, designed to explain why it is different organisations appear to be organised in similar ways, and how organisational innovation is diffused and institutional changes come about. The coercive variety, as its name suggests, results from external pressures from other organisations on which they are dependent. The obvious example is the role governments play in establishing regulatory frameworks within which health care organisations have to function. Mimetic isomorphism is commonly a response to uncertainty. For example, as the UK (Chapter 4) and Sweden (Chapter 3) became increasingly concerned about the rising costs of health care they, it might be suggested, adopted NPM even though it was unproven; it provided a legitimate response to uncertainty and offered the possibility that it might control costs while delivering services acceptable to the users. The normative variant refers to the assumed growing consensus around organisational norms as a consequence of the increasing professionalisation of the workforce, with the emphasis on university qualifications and membership of professional associations both underpinning an emphasis on normative behaviour (that is, acting professionally).

While this model is a useful one it does have limitations and its very logic involves overlooking some important features of organisations. As Morgan (1990:125) has usefully pointed out:

> there remains a gap between the myth of 'institutional isomorphism' and the actual situation within... organizations. This gap derives from two features. First, there is the power–knowledge dialectic identified by Foucault as a dynamic process where resistance/non-compliance continually arises... Second, there is the continued existence of alternative bases of organizational legitimation.

Hospitals are characterised precisely by these two features. For instance, physicians' knowledge base and professional status (legimacy) ensures their separate collective (professional) identity alongside their organisational membership of a hospital or clinic and they will resist reforms that threaten their professional autonomy. Nevertheless, despite reservations, what the New Institutionalism framework does offer is the opportunity, as Kitchener (1998:73–4) explains, to break out of the 'insular and parochial' disciplinary boundaries of much work on public sector organisations. The work situation[2] of health professionals can usefully be viewed as being part of an organisational field. This will include a range of institutions and organisations that coalesce to form a framework within which to understand inter- and intra- professional, management–professional and state–professional relations as well as patients and other consumers and users of the professionals' services. In addition, the field will include key suppliers such as the influential pharmaceutical companies.

It is equally possible and useful to examine organisational fields in terms of 'actor network theory' (ANT) for this approach shares some of the qualities of Foucauldian post-structuralism (Clegg 1989:202–7; Law 1992:387, 1994:18–21), which would permit greater integration with the model of professionalism presented earlier. Moreover, this particular standpoint has the advantage of bringing back into the analysis the matter of power relations, for ANT treats 'power as a (concealed or misrepresented) *effect*, rather than power as a set of causes' (Law 1992:387). This is a distinction that echoes Foucault's (1981) proposition: 'power is exercised from innumerable points, in the interplay of non-egalitarian and mobile relations' (Foucault, 1981:94) and reflects the dynamic processes by which actors become enmeshed – *enrolled* (Callon, 1986) – into a network. It is the means by which 'actors' and 'actants' have the possibility of resolving antagonisms and forming coalitions in order to establish a network of control (see also Clegg 1989:204). By contrast, the principal proponents of new institutionalism (see DiMaggio and Powell 1991a:22–6) own preference is to maintain some distinction between macro- and micro-levels of analysis preferring to draw on Giddens's (1984) notion of 'structuration' and Bourdieu's (1977) theory of *habitus*. The attraction, however, of translating New Institutionalism in a way compatible with ANT (see Clegg 1989:206), is that it enables one to adopt a position of empirical realism coupled with ontological relativism (Lee and Hassard 1999:393–4), a position that distinguishes it from both 'modern' and 'postmodern' analyses (Latour 1993:138–42) and provides a way around the challenges of actor/system dualism that faces new institutionalism without slipping into unbounded relativism.

Having set out the relevance and usefulness of the concept of organisational field it will now be useful to interrogate certain other New Institutionalism concepts that this analysis of comparative European hospital organisations and the medical and nursing professions relies upon. These are primarily 'archetypes', 'decoupling' and 'sedimentation'.

Organisational and professional legitimacy

In subordinating the concept of organisation to that of 'field' the new institutionalists claim that organisations can be best conceived as 'loosely coupled arrays of standardized elements' (DiMaggio and Powell 1991a:14) or 'archetypes' (Greenwood and Hinings 1993). Archetypes are ideal types and organisational change, for example, in the case of the introduction of NPM into health care organisations, can be conceptualised as a shift from one archetype to another. There are parallels here with 'path dependency' (Wilsford 1994) although that approach has the advantage of being much more self-consciously historical in assuming that later events – such as adapting to NPM – will be shaped by the earlier ones.[3] The elements of an archetype can be summarised in terms of, first, the 'interpretive scheme' or core values; second, 'systems' of control (strategic, financial and operational); and finally, 'structure' (differentiation and integration) (Greenwood and Hining 1993). Movement between archetypes, however, is not best understood as a linear process but conceptualised, as Cooper *et al.* (1996:624) have argued, dialectically:

> The basic argument is that organizational change represents not so much a shift from one archetype to another, but a layering of one archetype on another, Further, and to extend the geological analogy, what is exposed at the surface of the organization is the result of

a complex and historical process of faults and disruptions...
erosions...and strengths of the archetype.

This is a process of 'sedimentation', which allows for greater recognition
of the role of earlier practices, relations and conflicts to influence later
ones. Adopting this metaphor of sedimentation one can conceive of an
organisation manifesting more than one 'archetype' – or configuration –
as practices associated with earlier archetypes continue to co-exist with
that of later ones, figuratively, in the same way as in geology an older
rock stratum may well break through to the surface of later sedimenta-
tions. This also has a close resemblance to conceiving of organisations
in terms of an actor network for '[o]rganisations are in constant flux, and
different archetypes can dominate in different parts of the organization'
(ibid.: 635). This appears to be particularly true of hospitals being
formally reconfigured from professionally dominated to managerially
dominated organisations. This interpretation also has similarities to the
very useful notion of decoupling.

Meyer and Rowan's (1991:41) argue that the 'formal structures of
many organizations...reflect the myths of their institutional environ-
ments instead of the demands of their work activities'. There is, according to their argument, a 'decoupling' of the formal organisation 'myth'
from the reality (ibid.:57–8), which acts as an uncertainty-absorbing
arrangement that contributes to the legitimacy of an organisation and
its survival. A good example of 'decoupling' within any health system is
the exercise of clinical judgement. Doctors (physicians) are usually able
to follow the formal rules because these do not encompass in any
detail this discrete area of autonomy within the clinic (Harrison 1999).
Crucially, this 'decoupling' is not simply another way of classifying
the 'informal organisation'; it instead identifies the ambiguous nature
of professional, or specialist, judgement (discretion). Meyer and Rowan
(1991) argue that 'decoupling' of this kind is part of the means by which
complex organisations may function efficiently as well as legitimately,
which would otherwise be impossible. It is a similar concept to that of
'loose coupling' suggested by Weick (1976) and both provide the theoretical space to recognise the role knowledge/power discourses play
within organisations. Hospital doctors and nurses commonly have an
allegiance to their professional associations, an interest in their patients
and students and, possibly, the management of the hospital within
which they work. These interests can and do conflict. But if organisations are only 'loosely coupled' how do the actors play out their 'parts'
in such a way that an organisation can function in any way effectively?

Barley and Tolbert (1997:98) may provide a way of explaining how this process works. They draw on structuration theory (Giddens 1984) to underpin their analysis of the process by which actors adopt and adapt organisational scripts and in the process modify and reproduce institutions. The notion of scripts is drawn from the earlier work of one of the authors' (Barley 1986), which substitutes for Gidden's 'modalities'. These scripts are *'observable, recurrent activities and patterns of interaction characteristic of a particular setting'* (ibid.:98, emphases in original). This concept forms the basis of the 'four moments' of the institutionalisation process (Barley and Tolbert 1997:100–3), which can be summarised as follows:

1 'encoding of institutional principles in the scripts used in specific settings' (a socialisation and internalisation process);
2 enactment of the 'scripts that encode institutional principles' (which 'may or may not entail conscious choice');
3 revising or replicating scripts (intentional alteration 'is more likely to lead to institutional change' than those which are made unconsciously); and
4 'objectification and externalisation of the patterned behaviours and interactions produced during the period in question'

The sequence indicates how social actors construct scripts that then become institutionalised but, equally, provide the means of institutional change. It is very important to emphasise that the four moments of encoding, enactment, revision and objectification are ongoing processes: 'institutionalization...is a continuous process whose operation can be observed only through time' (Barley and Tolbert 1997:100). Changes are most likely to occur as a result of conscious intent and in response to changes in the wider environment (ibid.:102). A sense of continuity is commonly retained, it is assumed, because social interaction, within an organisational field, is 'constrained by histories and ritualistic patterning' (Barley 1986:107) and this leads to cumulative structuring and hence institutionalisation of new arrangements.

Barley and Tolbert define institutions as comprising of *'shared rules and typifications that identify categories of social actors and their appropriate activities or relationships'* (1997: 96, emphases in the original) and thereby avoids the reification of the notion of institution (see Berger and Luckman 1967:106–9). The aim is to construct a heuristic that takes account of the processual and embedded character of the 'structuration' of institutions and action (ibid.:96–7). This is a model that has parallels with the ANT approach discussed earlier but it is rooted in Gidden's structuration theory. Possibly as a consequence of this desire to maintain a strict structuralist interpretation of a structurational approach Barley and Tolbert restrict scripts to 'behavioural regularities' only (ibid.:98) which is unnecessarily limiting, particularly in the case of cross-country comparative studies where similar practices may well be rooted in very different histories and cultural practices. They use the metaphor of grammar and speech to explain the relation of institutions to actions, the assumption being that 'every expression must conform to an underlying set of tacitly understood rules'. Grammar, however, is not the tacit body of rules these authors assume. It varies between different cultures and countries. To mix metaphors – and thereby avoid discussing complex linguistics (cf. Giddens 1987:74–80) – a metaphor based on music might work better. The 'grammar' of music may be modal, harmonic, based on twelve-tone rows or some other system altogether. Musical grammar has changed at different times and different musical grammars have been in play at the same time in the West. In short, there is a greater heterogeneity in the taken-for-granted character of institutionalisation than these authors allow for. Thus, while there are isomorphic pressures towards a 'new' public management, variations in, for example, political systems (for example, unitary or federal states) and governance, which in Europe comes down to variations of the *Reichsstaat* – Corporatist – model of Continental Europe or the Anglo-Saxon notion of 'public interest' (Pollitt and Bouckaert 2000:52–4). Moreover, these factors historically have shaped the professional organisation of medicine and nursing in different ways and in the process ensured the impact of isomorphic forces will vary between countries. Rather than a globalised and 'McDonaldised' organisational template, one finds across Europe much more of an NPM theme and variations and much of it contrapuntal.

Conclusions

Whatever the differences between the work situations of doctors and nurses, the introduction of a discourse of 'new' managerialism in European health care has signalled revisions of the organisational scripts for both groups of professionals across much of Europe. Ostensibly the new managerialism is intended to subordinate them or, at least, to get them to comply more readily with the efficiency imperatives of managerial rationality. However, the changed and changing relations between the professionals and managers may not have been simply one of role reversal: for the new 'scripts' are more complex, suggesting more a reconfiguration of professional autonomy than its subordination. Moreover, this new managerial order has not affected all European countries to anything like the same degree. Some would appear to quite immune to the contagion. Here Germany and Greece provide particularly interesting and contrasting examples (see Chapters 5 and 6). In the next four chapters the character of health management reforms across eight European countries is examined and the implications of those reforms for medicine and nursing are assessed.

3
The Netherlands and Sweden: Quality Control

Sweden has spent more than any other country in Europe on its public sector, at least until recently. Health care spending in 1987 stood at 8.6 per cent of GDP, although this had declined to 7.7 per cent by the mid 1990s according to the 1996 OECD Health Data (Kanavos and McKee, 1998:27). The Netherlands spent comparable proportions on health services: 8.1 per cent in 1987 rising to 8.8 per cent in 1995 (ibid.). By 1998, however, Sweden's health expenditure at 8.4 per cent (European Observatory – Sweden 2001:25) was nearly at the same level it was in the 1980s. While the proportion spent on health services appears similar, the organisation of the funding of these two countries' health systems is quite different. In terms of Esping-Andersen's (1990) typology, The Netherlands is an example of Conservative Corporatism and Sweden represents an example of a Social Democratic welfare regime. Yet, as Pollitt and Bouckaert (2000:61) have observed, despite their differences, '[they] share a general disposition towards consensual, often meso-corporatist styles of governance'. This of itself would make the comparison of the two countries' health systems and professional organisation interesting. But there are additional and possibly better reasons why they are particularly useful comparators with which to start this series of paired case studies (Chapters 3–6). First, both countries were early adopters of the 'quasi-market',[1] within the health care system. The Netherlands adopted the approach in 1987, earlier than any other country in Europe (Dekker 1987; Ham, Robinson and Benzeval 1990:44–5) with Sweden, introducing the principle during the period 1991–94 (Rehnberg 1997:68), more influenced by the UK than The Netherlands. Second, and relatedly, the issue of professional 'quality control' among hospital doctors has been approached differently in the two countries. The Netherlands's medical profession has been at the forefront of developing clinical guidelines within Europe in order, in part, to emphasise its autonomy from the state. By contrast, the Swedish medical profession has been happier to work closely with government in these developments. Both these issues (quasi-markets and clinical governance) have been key developments within European health care systems in the 1990s. It is true that the quasi-market has become less of a central issue, giving way to an even more managerialist and putatively New Public Management (NPM) agenda, with the issue of clinical guidelines and related notions of evidence-based medicine and care pathways continuing to grow in importance.

Another factor that influenced their selection for comparison was that they were both small countries in terms of relative population when compared to the larger European countries: Germany (82 million), Britain (58.8 million), Italy (57 million) and France (56.6 million). The Netherlands, by contrast, has a population of around 15.5 million (Eurostat 1996) and Sweden 8.9 million (WHO 2000c). There are, however, considerable demographic differences between these two Northern European countries. The Netherlands is a small, densely packed country located in Continental Europe with borders with two of the largest European countries, Germany and France, whereas Sweden covers a territory considerably larger than Britain with 85 per cent of its people living in its southern half.

The Netherlands and Sweden represent critical cases of European adoption and adaptation of health reforms for the following reasons. First, the changes grew out of, or were integrated into, their particular political, social and organisational cultures of their respective health systems. Second, the changes reflect the dynamic tension between the medical profession and the state. In The Netherlands the medical profession has always strongly insisted on its separateness from the state and the organisation of health care delivery whereas in Sweden the opposite has generally been the case. On the issue of nursing, what is presented here is the beginning of a discussion on the variations and commonalities of nursing across Europe that will be threaded through the subsequent chapters.

The chapter is organised in four sections. First, an overview of the two health systems, hospitals and their reforms, followed by a section that deals with the medical profession and the issue of clinical governance. A comparison of the nursing professions and hospital work comes next, followed by a short concluding section for the chapter as a whole.

The health systems, hospitals and the reforms in Netherlands and Sweden

Both countries were early adopters of the principles of the quasi-market, or regulated market, as promoted by Enthoven (1978, 1985, 1989; Harrison and Calltorp 2000:220). Although the influence would appear to have been less direct than in the case of the UK and it has been argued, in the case of The Netherlands, that 'there is no direct evidence that [the reforms] were based on the economic theories of Alain Enthoven [at all]' (Björkman and Okma 1997:94), whether this was the case or not there is sufficient similarity to justify the adoption of the term 'regulated' or 'quasi-market'. These two countries very usefully demonstrate the importance of not overgeneralising the impact of institutional isomorphism for, despite drawing on common quasi-market thinking, the initial health systems were differently organised (drawing on different traditions) (Jacobs 1998), the trajectory followed was different (see Pollitt and Bouckaert 2000:62–3) and consequently the outcomes were not the same either. The purpose of this section is to present and explain these differences – this convergence on parallel lines – starting with the case of The Netherlands.

The Netherlands

Historical context

The Netherlands' health system was historically shaped by the pillarisation (*verzuiling*) of society. This peculiarly Dutch institutional arrangement, formally established in the early part of the twentieth century, has effectively enabled Catholic, Protestant and secularist interests to co-exist within a coalition of social solidarity (Smith 1988:172). It is therefore the organisations representing these interests (particularly labour unions and employers associations) that have dictated the role of the state that, in turn, is recognised as the representative of the public interest – subject to the prior autonomy of particular interest groups. Catholics call this principle 'subsidiarity', the Protestants 'sovereignty'. The Dutch government, however, is not without power, for it has responsibility for balancing out the various claims within what is known as the 'middle field' (*Maatschappelijk middenveld*) in order to represent a consociational public interest (Björkman and Okma 1997:80). This has particular implications for the organisation and reform of health care, not least because within this framework the medical profession has a high degree of autonomy.

The financing of health care has been primarily from social and private health insurance, which under the Sickness Fund Act (ZFW) of 1964 meant that about 60 per cent of the Dutch population were enrolled with one of the 25 sickness funds (Björkman and Okma 1997:81). The remaining population were mostly privately insured, with civil servants being provided with their own insurance scheme. Subscribers' premiums were set at a uniform percentage of gross income. The sickness funds concluded contracts with health care providers (for example, hospitals) on behalf of their subscribers. Until 1992 sickness funds had no discretion over what hospitals or clinics they contracted with; instead the terms were negotiated nationally. In addition, there was a specific insurance, implemented in 1967, to cover long-term care. This was known as the Exceptional Medical Expenses Act (AWBZ) and employers paid these premiums as a percentage of employees' wages. Those not covered by sickness fund or insurance (for example, the unemployed or elderly) had their health care cost covered directly by government.

Dekker and the quasi-market

All this changed in the wake of the Dekker Committee, set up in 1986 and reporting the following year (Ham, Robinson and Benzeval 1990:44). This committee was set up in the wake of the failure of a previous reform programme of cost containment the principles of which were contained in the 'Memorandum on the Structure of Health Care' (VOMIL 1974) which was widely experienced as too bureaucratic and centralised. There is a similarity here to the experience of Swedish experience of the Dagmar reforms a decade later (see below). One consequence was a widespread disbelief in the ability of any bureaucratic system to bring about cost containment which was seen as politically and organisationally too cumbersome. The main features of the Dekker report can be summarised in three points.

1 Radical restructuring of the sickness fund and private health insurance system with the introduction of a single basic insurance scheme covering 85 per cent of costs. On top of this there would be an optional, supplementary, insurance for those services not otherwise covered (for example, dental care, medicines and physiotherapy).
2 Simplification of the payment system. The basic insurance contributions would be paid as an income-related premium deducted from the employee's wage or salary. The supplementary insurance would be paid as a flat-rate premium directly to the insurance company of choice.

3 There would be an overt shift to regulation by the market and a clear move away from regulation by directives to regulation by incentives. This, it was believed, would lead to competition between 'purchasers' (insurance companies) and 'providers' (for example, hospitals) and thereby to greater efficiency. This is the classic 'steering not rowing' strategy advocated by Osborne and Gaebler (1992) a few years later.

This introduction of a quasi-market was the outcome of a political consensus among all the main political parties that cost containment within health care could no longer be solely the responsibility of government. In future it was to be shared with the health insurers and sickness funds (Schut 1995:72). However, in order for this to be achieved it would be necessary to introduce a level playing field within this new and competitive (quasi-)market. Hence the sickness funds became health insurers in their own right with the freedom for the first time to enter into contracts with providers selectively. The insurers' incentive lay in contracting with only the more efficient providers, thus holding down costs and thereby maximising their profits (Ham, Robinson and Benzeval 1990:45). Health insurance premiums, however, have been based on a simple capitation formula of age, sex and location. This has the advantage of reducing the management costs as well as dealing with the issue of how to ensure that high-risk groups would not be disadvantaged and that the insurance companies would not disproportionately concentrate on 'cream skimming' the low-risk cases (Van de Ven and Van Vliet 1997). The formula is not able, to provide the opportunity for efficiency saving, however (Schut 1995:79–80). The providers incentive would be to find economies over and beyond those reflected in the prospective contract payments. Part of this process has led to a greater emphasis being put on primary care and integrated care packages, as well as substitution of inpatient care by ambulatory care in the policlinic (Harrison and Lieverdink 2000:72). In the longer term the aim has been to reduce the number of beds and close the less efficient hospitals. It was intended that this would promote the development of HMO[2]-type organisations and thereby improve efficiencies and quality of the health services (Ham, Robinson and Benzeval, 1990:45).

While the original Dekker recommendations had widespread political support, implementation proved difficult. This has been partly because changing governing coalitions meant different emphases to the reform programme. The Christian Democrats favoured more the free enterprise elements while the Social Democrats were more committed to the egalitarian elements of the programme. Nevertheless, the generality of the Dekker reforms did take root. There does appear to have been a consensus around the central assumption that, in pursuing their legitimate self-interest and responsibilities, players in the market would create a virtuous circle of continuous improvements in efficiency and quality. The particular players with which I am concerned here are the hospitals and the medical and nursing professions.

Hospitals and specialists

There are around 143 general (acute) teaching and specialised hospitals ranging from small, 100 bed, to very large 1100 bed institutions (Berg and van der Grinten forthcoming). Some 90 per cent of Dutch hospitals are charitable, not-for-profit institutions, typically of religious origins and reflecting a fundamental corporatist principle of subsidiarity that 'what can be handled in the private sphere should not be undertaken by government' (ibid.). There are around 13,000 hospital specialists (ibid.) the majority (about 90 per cent) being paid on a 'fee for service' basis and only 10 per cent are salaried. This includes doctors working within university hospitals, psychiatrists and paediatricians. According to *The Netherlands: Nursing and Midwifery Profile* (WHO 1994)[3] there is one doctor per 315 persons. Patients are referred to hospital specialists from general practice, where there the ratio is 1:2325 GPs per head of population. Within the hospital system itself the hospital specialists successfully blocked all, or most, of the reforms relating to their income and employment status as well as to their direct involvement in hospital management (Harrison and Lieverdink 2000:68). Nevertheless, the Government remained committed to a policy of reducing and integrating hospital specialists' earnings into hospitals' budgets rather than their being treated as separate.

In 1993 the Secretary for Health (Simons) initiated a substantial cut of 12 per cent for most specialist fees and even more for the highest earning specialties. The general policy was given a further push by the Biesheuvel Report in 1994 which recommended that hospital specialists should be paid a salary-type income – more accurately, a prospective payment system based on expected workloads. The reforms were intended to encourage hospitals (and doctors) to compete to provide good-quality care at a competitive price. In order to achieve this goal the reforms advocated the participation of specialists in the management and the replacement of the inflationary 'fee for service' (FFS) system of payment (van de Ven 1997:97). The Dutch doctors, however, proved themselves very attached to the FFS system and the issue divided the medical specialists association (LSV) and led to the establishment of the breakaway Netherlands Specialist Federation (NSF) (Schut 1995:69;

Harrison and Lieverdink 2000:67–8). This group rejoined LSV in 1997. The consistency of the Government in seeking to incorporate hospital specialists' incomes within the hospitals' budgets and thereby bring them within the broader 'managed care' frame is really quite impressive. The importance of the Biesheuvel Committee's report here is that it was telling the medical profession that they had to compromise with the Government over earnings and hospital management or they would lose even more autonomy and income via more draconian measures. Moreover, following the election of the left of centre 'purple coalition' in 1994, the Government had the necessary political and public support outside to achieve this. The then new Minister of Health (Mrs Borst-Eiler) offered a guarantee to maintain specialists' earnings level for three years for those who co-operated and a policy of threatened fee cuts for those who did not (Harrison and Lieverdink 2000:69). In January 1998 the Netherland's two Houses of Parliament accepted the amendment that integrated medical fees into hospital finances.

The politics of this process was at times quite Byzantine. Hospital specialists threatened with direct control by management, have begun to come around to accepting the need to be involved in hospital management and, possibly, to accepting a prospective and collective 'fees for services' method of calculating incomes (so long as it is not called a salary). This approach would protect the specialists' strong belief in their entrepreneurialism and their role as independent medical providers. But, and this is the key, it will also enable the health insurance organisations (as purchasers) to operate within a known cost structure. The implementation of the scheme was only possible subject to a government promise of exemption from income reductions for those doctors willing to participate. Even so, most specialists have not become involved in these 'partnership in management' experiments outside the approximately seventy participating hospitals. Instead, specialists' incomes are now, in effect, capped in a way that parallels the practice in Germany (see Chapter 5), the capping although is imposed by the hospital management and not the 'doctors' chambers' (*Ärtzekammer*). Once the budget for a particular service or specialty has been spent, and this includes the funds for specialists' FFS incomes, no more patients are treated until new funds are available (Berg 2001). The willingness of The Netherlands's doctors to become involved in hospital reforms, therefore, must never be overstated. The situation in Sweden is rather different in that the hospital specialists have not seen themselves as entrepreneurial in any sense; instead, their professional autonomy has been very closely intertwined with administrative responsibilities.

Sweden

Historical context

Swedish health care has been in the public sector for nearly five hundred years (Garpenby 1992:19). Following the establishment of the county councils in 1862 the health services increasingly became their responsibility. Jumping ahead to 1944[4] and the publication of *Post-war Programme of the Workers' Movement* (*Arbetarrörelsons Efterkrigsprogram*), more prosaically known as: 'The Twenty-seven Points' ('De 27 Punkterna'), setting out the fundamental reforms for the establishment of the Swedish Welfare State, which was published jointly by the Social Democratic Party (SDP) and the union organisation (*Landsorganisationen i Sverige*). The reforms were successfully implemented because, basically, the SDP was in a strong position politically, a period known in Sweden as the SDP's 'harvest time'.

The reforms meant that the system of health care was to be based on a national health insurance scheme. This was introduced with broad political support in 1947 although there were misgivings on the part of the white-collar workers' union (TCO) and the Swedish Employers' Federation (SAF). The strength of electoral support for the reforms, however, was so strong that neither group overtly opposed the reforms. Nevertheless, the pace of change was slow. Regional government was at that time reluctant to spend too much money too fast (Garpenby 2002). In 1948, however, it looked as if the SDP might be just too radical. In that year the Höjer Commission (chaired by the director of the National Board of Health) reported and recommended a fundamental transformation of the organisation and delivery of health care. Particular attention was paid to reorganising nationally the system of outpatient care, which was then under the control of the country councils.

The proposals also recommended that medical staff should be salaried in future rather than being paid 'fee for service' (as was then the norm) and all private practice within the public sector hospitals would be prohibited. Unlike 'The Twenty-seven Points this report engendered much hostile opposition even, perhaps surprisingly, from the county councils. One concern was that these proposed reforms would drive all (or most) doctors into private practice, leaving the public hospitals and outpatients clinics (*polikliniks* or *Primärvården*)[5] without a viable medical workforce. Another even more fundamental concern was whether the future Swedish health service would be a primary care based one as Höjer intended or one based on and around large acute hospitals (Garpenby 2002). The political pressure became so great that the proposals came to be seen as unworkable and the reform was dropped.

The 'Seven Crowns' reforms

It took another twenty years before what is often seen as the essential elements of the Swedish health system were introduced. The changes are known as the 'Seven Crowns (Kronor)' reforms and were introduced in 1969 designed to make health care more accessible to low-income groups (European Observatory – Sweden 2001:8). The 'Seven Kronor' refers to the proposed minimal charge (co-payment), which approximated to a little less than $10 (US) at the time for visiting an outpatient clinic (*poliklinik*). At the same time the county councils would be paid 31 Kronor from the national health insurance for each visit. One of the intended and realised outcomes was that private practice virtually 'dried up'. Patients could still visit a private practitioner after 1969 under the health insurance arrangements, but they would only receive 75 per cent reimbursement (Immergut 1992) so, given the choice of either paying just seven crowns or paying the much higher fees for visiting an office (private) physician, patients were quick to opt for the less expensive option. The pricing mechanism virtually dried up the private market for health care and effectively closed the door to any doctor wanting to exit the public sector by that route or even simply to supplement his or her income. The county council this time, unlike in 1948, supported the changes. The medical profession, however, was divided: senior members of the profession, particularly those working in large hospitals, were against the changes while younger hospital doctors and those working in rural practice were supportive.[6] The salaries on offer were attractive enough to these groups, whose chances for earning substantial amounts from private practice was in any case quite limited.

The quasi-market reforms

In the early 1990s a quasi-market was introduced into the health care system. The policy was crucially influenced by the work of Enthoven (1989); Axelsson (2000:50); Harrison and Calltorp (2000:220) particularly as they had been implemented in Britain (Whitehead, Gustafsson, and Diderichsen 1997:935). The reforms were introduced in part because the previous policy of cost control through tight budgetary constraints in the 1980s had been too successful (Saltman 1990:597). It had been the Dagmar Reforms of 1985 that had given the county councils far-reaching responsibility for reforming health care delivery. At that time the political consensus was firmly behind a planned, social democratic, approach to health care policy and delivery. Confidence in this approach, however, had slipped by the late 1980s because the success of this policy of cost-containment (using global budgets) deprived the service of resources and skilled people and led to longer waiting lists with the consequence that the tiny private health care sector was showing clear signs of growth.[7] These concerns, coupled with a lack of any alternative ideas (that is, a prima facie case of mimetic isomorphism) led to the adoption of market-oriented mechanisms (Saltman 1990:598; Whitehead *et al.* 1997:935; Axelsson 2000:50; Harrison and Calltorp 2000:220). However, the adoption of the quasi-market within Swedish health care was quite different from that in The Netherlands.

The first key difference was that in Sweden the quasi-market was introduced locally and experimentally by the county councils (and municipalities)[8]–not by central government (Garpenby 1992; Saltman and Von Otter 1992; Rehnberg 1997:68–70). Even so, central government did put regional government under pressure to reform the organisation of health care services, not least by tax changes that favoured central government and reduced funding to the regions (Garpenby 2002). Right from the start the policy was as much about decentralisation as it was about markets. There were a number of variations, but basically there were three main models tried (Rehnberg 1997:69).

1 *Dala model*. These county councils (Dalarna, Bohuslän) decentralised purchasing to primary health districts with populations of 6,000–50,000.
2 *Stockholm model*. These include Stockholm and Västerbotten and organised around larger purchasing boards than in the Dala model.
3 *Centralised model*. Some county councils have set up central agencies to act as the collective purchaser for all citizens (Sörmland, Östergötland).

It was, according to Whitehead *et al.*, (1997:936) 'only in Stockholm County, however, that the reforms go as far as a managed market system introducing competition between provider'.

Even so, the reforms elsewhere were influenced directly by quasi-market thinking. The second difference was that the reforms were generally welcomed (or not opposed) at the local level. As several commentators have observed, for example, local politicians saw the internal market as a way of improving their image (that had suffered under the cost containment policy) as the representatives of the citizens' health care interests as members of the county council purchaser boards (Garpenby 1992:24). The doctors, similarly, saw the changes in a positive light, even if they '[were] inexperienced in how to behave in a competitive environment' (ibid.:17). A third difference, when compared to The Netherlands, was the apparent creation of markets *internal* to the hospitals when clinical budgets were introduced in the 1980s. Clinical departments were financed by activity-based revenues rather than fixed budgets (Wiley 1998:231). This system was based on the principle that the more work a department carried out the more money it 'earned'; furthermore, the dynamic of this process would improve their efficiency. One of the problems with the approach turned out to be that the arrangements appeared to systematically favoured radiology, laboratory and similar service departments, for they would earn all the revenues from providing services to the clinical departments that required those services. The particular Swedish mix of decentralised health care delivery coupled with the social democratic ethos shaped those reforms. Equally relevant, however, has been the long-established incorporation of the medical profession, which can mean that Swedish doctors appear, even to themselves, more like civil servants than autonomous professionals. They work fixed hours, on salaries and, unlike the case of The Netherlands' medical profession there is little separation between medical and managerial responsibilities within hospitals. Senior doctors manage *qua* manage departments and hospitals and have done so for a long time (Lane and Arvidson 1989:92–3). The introduction of quasi-market reforms was not seen as contentious by the profession (Garpenby 1992:19) and some even welcomed the reforms as a means of providing a basis for a new professional autonomy independent of the state (ibid.:17).

Both The Netherlands and Sweden had, by the mid 1990s, seen a slowdown in the reforms, and the policy analysts started to look to more managerialist solutions to controlling costs and ensuring quality (Harrison and Calltorp 2000:220; Axelsson 2000:50). One line of development that took root during the quasi-market reform period was the quality of care. Sweden in particular had established arrangements for ensuring public confidence in the quality of hospital care while the medical profession in The Netherlands were early adopters of consensus clinical guidelines. Nevertheless, the introduction of the quasi-market within both countries did also directly influence quality of care issues and policies in ways that went beyond the contractual relations of purchasers and providers. Before examining this set of issues in any detail, however, it will first be useful to provide an account of the two medical professions, for quality of care is always the claim of the medical profession as part of its claim to autonomy. Increasingly, however, this claim has to be transparent and inclusive of other social actors and agencies. The question arises, are the current generation of quality controls on medicine eroding doctors' autonomy? Before answering it is necessary to point out in the case of Sweden (unlike The Netherlands) the dynamic nature of the relations between central government and the county councils.

Government, county councils and health care

Within the Swedish system of administration there is a dynamic tension between central government and the county councils. Health care has been a particularly contested terrain at least since the mid 1970s. The National Board of Health and Welfare (NBHW) (*Socialstyrelsen*) has taken the more centralist view while the Federation of County Councils (FCC) (*Landstingsförbundet*) have advocated a decentralist policy. With the introduction of the quasi-market they were ultimately successful and, even after the marketisation elements of the policy began to wane in the mid 1990s following the re-election of the Social Democrats, the decentralist policy remained in place. Nevertheless, according to Garpenby (1999:411), what the Ministry of Health and Social Affairs strives for is a 'creative conflict' at the national level in order, in part, to be able to influence local government politicians and health care provider organisations. To this end, the Ministry relies on the relations between the NBHW and the FCC.

Hospitals and specialists

There are approximately 30,000 doctors working in Sweden providing a ratio of 1:296.7 population (WHO 2000c:5,12). Most of these doctors will be hospital specialists as the health system is very much a hospital-orientated system. General practice has not played a significant role within the health care system and there had long been a shortage of GP provision across Sweden (Garpenby 1992:22). In the early 1990s, for instance, there were approximately 24,000 medical doctors in Sweden (21,000 in the public sector) of which only 2,500 were GPs. Patients, it appears, much preferred to use the *poliklinik* services, and only since the late 1990s has a GP referral been required.

Sweden has about 79 hospitals divided into regional, central county and district county hospitals (European Observatory – Sweden 2001:55). The country is divided into six medical care regions each serving a population of between 1 and 2 million people. These are responsible for the country's nine highly specialised regional hospitals, which also function as research and teaching hospitals (eight are affiliated to university medical schools). These hospitals provide the full range of specialist care and are administered by the county within which they are located and regulated by agreement between the county councils within the region.

Central government contributes for the costs for teaching and research. These hospitals deal with complex cases referred from other hospitals as well as providing secondary care to the local population. The next level of hospital care is provided by the 23 central county hospitals (one for each county council area), with 15–20 specialties, that serve as the district hospital for the geographical area. These are administered by the county councils, as are the 47 smaller 'district county hospitals' with at least four specialties of internal medicine, surgery, radiology and anesthesiology able to deliver basic acute services.

Professional organisation of medicine and clinical governance

Professional organisation

The principal difference between the medical professions of the two countries is that The Netherlands' profession views its autonomy as reflecting its independence from the state and the management of the hospitals while their Swedish counterparts do not. Their ascendant position within the Swedish health care system has lain precisely in their commitment to working within the public sector aided by the Social Democratic Government's expansion of medical posts during the 1970s (Garpenby 2002).

The medical profession in The Netherlands

The Netherlands Medical Association (NMG) was officially established in 1849 (Klazinga 1996:77). Their members were mostly general practitioners and an independent specialist association was only founded much later in 1910 and incorporated into the NMG in 1914. In 1931 a specialist register was established and post-graduate training formalised. In 1946 the Dutch Specialist Association (LSV) was established as a component part of the NMG alongside the Dutch Association for Family Doctors (LHV). The NMG became 'Royal' in 1949 (KNMG). Alongside these developments groups of specialists organised scientific societies, in much the same way as elsewhere in Europe. The first of these was the Scientific Society of Psychiatry and Neurology founded in 1873, the Society of Surgery was established in 1902 while the Society of Medicine did not come into being until 1931 (ibid.:104). In addition, local professional associations were founded; unlike the scientific societies these were concerned with the economic interests of their members.

The hospital specialists enjoy considerable professional dominance and autonomy which is rooted in the institutionalisation of the 'closed hospital' policy established in the decades following the Second World War (ibid.:80–2). The closed hospital policy meant specialists having exclusive contracts with only one hospital. However, organisationally within that hospital the specialists were able to maintain wholly separate billing arrangements. They operated as a wholly independent body within the hospital. They were – and remain – organised in 'partnerships' (*maatschappen*), which further reinforced their autonomy.

[a *maatschap*] is a partnership of medical specialists of the same medical discipline. Apart from the defence of its joint financial interests within the hospital (fees...are pooled and divided...among members), such a partnership plays a role in the co-ordination of clinical activities and in introduction of medical innovations. (Schepers and Casparie 1997:597)

The individual *maatschappen* are represented on the Medical Staff Committee, a body with no direct link into strategic hospital management yet retaining much influence through the work of the Medical Staff Committee, which not only represents the interests of the doctors but also takes – or claims – the responsibility for the co-ordination of the work of the nursing and other health professionals. This reflects a practical co-existence between management and medicine '[of a] peculiar combination of separation and integration...[in which] hospital management and medical specialists are bound up within one hospital organisation...[but] not bound in a hierarchical relation' (Berg and van der Grinten, forthcoming). This configuration of 'loosely coupled' arrangements is rooted in the strongly embedded professional values of Dutch doctors that they, as free professionals, are the entrepreneurs that provide the work and income for the hospital and other professionals. The case of Sweden is rather different.

The Swedish medical profession

The Collegium Medicum dates back to 1663 and the Surgical Society was incorporated in 1797. In 1813 the Collegium Medicum voluntarily allowed itself to be replaced by the Health College which in 1877 became the National Board of Health (*Medicinalstyrelsen*) and the National Board of Health and Welfare (*Socialstyrelsen*) in 1968 (Garpenby 1992:19–20; Immergut 1992:187–8). It is the SSM (*Svenska läkaresällskapet*) and the SMA (*Sveriges läkarförbund*) who are the independent components of the Swedish medical profession. The Swedish Society of Medicine (SSM) is a scientific society established in 1808 which zealously avoids all involvement with economic issues (Immergut 1992: 188). These latter matters are handled by the doctors' trade union, the Swedish Medical Association (SMA) which currently represents well over 90 per cent of the doctors (Garpenby, 1999:410). It is the medical faculties at the universities which have the dominant position within the SSM. The body is primarily concerned with medical research and education as well as the issue of standards and accountability. It deals directly with the state, in the form of the NBHW or the Ministry of Health at national level. The real power of this organisation lies with the highly autonomous specialty associations of which there are more than sixty. The largest of these represent general practice, general surgery and internal medicine (Garpenby 1999:410). The SMA is, by contrast, much more democratic. Membership of the organisation is channelled through seven professional associations and 28 local associations[9] the largest of which is the Swedish Association of Hospital Physicians (*Sjukhusläkarföreningen*)[10] followed by the Swedish Junior Hospital Physicians Association. The SMA also deals extensively with the Federation of Country Councils on issues such as conditions of service and continuing education as well as with the Ministry over the formation of national policy. The Association also represents the profession on government consultation committees dealing with health care policy.

One of the key issues to have emerged from the quasi-market experience and to inform the development of managed care, which impinges directly on medical work has been that of quality, especially in the form of clinical guidelines. The Netherlands was an early adopter of guidelines while Sweden was not. The reasons for this are discussed in the following section.

Clinical governance

The term clinical governance is perhaps more widely used in the UK than in either of the two countries discussed here. Nevertheless, I wish to use the term to refer to a system of oversight designed to ensure good clinical practice. This may be achieved by a variety of means, but particularly influential during the 1990s and 2000s has been the use of clinical guidelines (or protocols). It is an innovation is of North American origin and one that was adopted and adapted uniquely by The Netherlands medical profession while initially being largely ignored in Sweden. How this came about and why is the purpose of this section of the chapter. In addition, the implications for changing the relations between the medical profession and management within both countries will be discussed. The argument presented is that the quality control of hospital care (including clinical guidelines) emerged on to centre stage as part of the long-standing and ongoing negotiations between state and the organised profession over professional and clinical autonomy. The adoption of quasi-market solutions within The Netherlands and Sweden reflected a broader movement to reconfigure European health care delivery systems in ways that provided (for the state) a more efficient system with little or no erosion of the principle of equity (for example Ham 1997:130). Part of the rhetoric of a regulated market was that it provided consumer choice and promised customer satisfaction, and this became the watchword for quality management generally. From the perspective of the medical profession, while patient satisfaction is important even more so is the effectiveness of the care and treatment in the light of current scientific and clinical knowledge.

The medical profession within The Netherlands was probably the first in Europe to adopt and widely implement a version of clinical guidelines. The particular institutionalised form that the quality control of clinical practice takes within a particular health care system is primarily shaped by three interrelated elements within the field: (1) recent history of profession/state relations; (2) pre-existing arrangements for quality control; (3) acceptability of managerial systems of quality management.

In the following sections these aspects will be discussed in relation first to The Netherlands and then Sweden.

The Netherlands

In wake of the Dekker report the Royal Dutch Medical Association (KNMG) organised a government-sponsored conference in 1989 (and again in 1990 and 1995) held in Leidschendam (near The Hague) with the aim of establishing a national quality care policy (Casparie 1993; Klazinga 1996:94). It was not only doctors who attended this conference for hospital managers, representatives of the patients' associations and the sickness funds also participated (government officials attended as observers). One aim of the conference was to put in place quality assurance systems that would meet the WHO recommendations mentioned earlier. Another was to ensure that contracting between purchasers and providers would include the quality of services as well as patients' (users') concerns in addition to volume and price (Klazinga 1996:94). There were three central concerns to be addressed:

1 to assure good quality of care in the absence of direct government regulation
2 to ensure that cost containment was not at the expense of quality of care
3 to counteract any tendency on the part of insurance companies (sickness funds) to disadvantage particular groups of patients (for example, those with chronic diseases or serious disabilities).

The outcome was an agreement over the role the different parties would play in quality assurance. Providers would be principally responsible for quality of care; purchasers would ensure the efficiency and organisation of care; while the patient organisations would review the culture of care (Casparie 1993:139). This approach reflected the traditional corporatist (consultative and consensual) political culture of The Netherlands. The problem in adopting this consociational approach, however, was that implementing and monitoring the agreements locally was a complex process. Within two years of the first conference more than half the 23 scientific associations had introduced peer review although only three had adopted external review. Most adopted the use of consensus clinical guidelines. Neither the insurance companies nor the patients' associations became actively involved in any quality assurance initiatives. The Government underpinned the agreement with a bill on quality of care demanding all health institutions set up internal quality systems and publish annual reports on their quality assurance policy.

The Leidschendam conferences were not the first time introduction of quality assurance had been debated within the Dutch health care system. The medical profession had established their National Organisation for Peer Review in Hospitals (CBO) back in 1976 (Reerink 1990; Casparie 1995:557). The CBO started work on the consensus development of explicit clinical criteria in 1982 and produced 39 sets of guidelines a decade later (Klazinga 1994:56–7). The attraction of this approach to the hospital specialists was that they perceived it as less burdensome than the system of hospital-based peer review (medical audit). Collectively they preferred to rationalise the system by adopting this national system of clinical guidelines organised by their professional associations (Casparie 1991:253). These guidelines were formulated as follows: a topic was selected, a chairperson appointed and experts recruited through their scientific societies. Typically an expert group would have ten members and meet monthly over a one-year period. The group would write up the background (technical) papers for discussion at a specially convened consensus conference of around three hundred participants. The final text would be published in a medical journal. The process was initially a wholly medical matter, but later representatives of the health insurers and patients associations began to be involved. Rather than representing an erosion of the doctors' autonomy, however, it would appear to be a price that the profession is willing to pay in order to maintain credibility with the general public. The difficulty with the approach, however, was that the profession was unable to demonstrate that the guidelines led to any measurable improvements. They may have done but the CBO appear to have lacked the techniques to direct measure what the benefits were. Nevertheless, the Dutch medical profession became adept at using the guidelines to both defend its autonomy and demonstrate their accountability towards the other groups.

Sweden

The Swedish case is rather different for reasons intimated earlier, namely, that the medical profession did not feel the need to develop clinical guidelines or take part in any new systems of clinical governance. In his study of medical quality assurance comparing and assessing progress towards the WHO (1985) target for quality assurance within European and US health care systems Jost (1990:68) commented, 'experts...believe that Sweden [is] lagging behind in developing quality assurance programmes, that many hospitals were lax in the area of quality assurance, and that the quality of care suffers because of this'. This is strong stuff. Yet it is the case that Swedish citizens, according to a *Eurobarometer* survey conducted in 1996 and reported in Mossialos (1997), have been well satisfied with their health system, with only 4.7 per cent recording dissatisfaction (Mossialos 1997), although in the more recent *Eurobarometer* reported in European Observatory – Sweden (2001:57) the level of dissatisfaction had risen to 26.1 per cent. This may well be a consequence of the cost containment policies implemented during the 1990s (ibid.). It is possible that Swedish doctors will come under greater pressure to adopt quality assurance although the public dissatisfaction with the health services may well be more related to access to the hospital specialist rather than their concerns about the quality of medical care delivered. Moreover, as Rehnberg (1997:65) points out, much of the good health enjoyed by Swedes is not the result of the health care system but rather it is attributable to the quality of housing, education and public health infrastructure. The result is that the general health of the population is good and, in terms of life expectancy, infant mortality and perinatal mortality, the statistics show

Sweden to be one of the healthiest places in the world (Abbott and Giarchi 1997:359–78 *passim*; European Observatory-Sweden 4–5). Against this background it is hardly surprising that there has been little pressure on the medical profession to prioritise quality of care programmes.

Another possible reason for an early lack of early interest in the introduction of a quality assurance system based on guidelines as in the case of The Netherlands was because there was already a well accepted and respected system of quality control in place, known as the *lex maria* (Rosenthal 1992, 2002), although the effectiveness of this system should not be overstated. This is a system whereby prima facie cases of medical mistakes have to be reported to the *Socialstyren* (National Board of Health and Welfare, NBHW) and dealt with by the Medical Responsibility Board (*Hälso-och Sjukvärdens Ansvarsnämnd*). This latter body is chaired by a judge and comprises of four members of *Riksdag*, three members of health care unions and a representative of the county councils. Only one the representative of the physicians union is likely to be a doctor. The MRBs workload covers all health professionals but most of its work involves doctors. A specialist doctor researches and presents the case as well as making recommendations of how it should be dealt with. Rosenthal (1992:42) reports that the doctors are 'disproportionately and consistently influential in the decision-making'. The majority of complaints (about 85 per cent) come from patients or their representatives and the remainder originate from the National Board of Health and Social Welfare, Parliamentary Ombudsman or the Office of the Chancellor of Justice (Jost 1990:30). The decisions of the MRB are made public.

Despite broad satisfaction with the health care system and public confidence in the health professionals the introduction of the quasi-market, decentralisation as well as the need to address the demands of the WHO (1985) to implement a comprehensive quality assurance programme all added up to a need for change. Garpenby (1999), in an article discussing the Swedish policy network in relation to quality control in health care, produced a useful diagram of the main organisations at national level involved in quality of health care in Sweden (see Figure 3.1) and which will be drawn upon here to provide this account of the roles of the main social actors.

National Board of Health and Welfare and Ministry of Health and Social Affairs.
At the national level it is the National Board of Health and Welfare (NBHW) that is responsible, under the Ministry of Health and Social

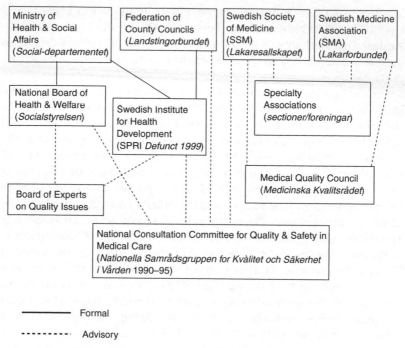

——————— Formal

- - - - - - - - - Advisory

Figure 3.1 Main organisations in the 'policy community' of quality in health care in Sweden
Source: Garpenby 1999:408

Affairs, for monitoring, follow-up and evaluation of health care.[11] This body has a great deal of autonomy in the way it carries out its responsibilities, which are set out by Government in the form of standing instructions and annual assignments. The NBHW came into being in 1968 following the merger of National Board of Health (*Medicalstyrelsen*) and the National Board of Social Affairs (*Socialstyrelsen*).

With the decentralisation of the health care system in the 1990s the role of central government in relation to quality issues changed in a quite distinct way. It now took on the task of watchdog and regulator in the delivery of health. The NBHW was mandated this task and specifically to compile outcome data, document good health care practice as well as more assiduously monitor hospitals, nursing homes and laboratories, and other licensed organisations (Garpenby 1999:409).

Federation of County Councils (FCC). During the 1980s there had been a tendency for the Federation of County Councils (FCC) (*Landstings-förbundet*) to compete with the NBHW and assume a quasi-authority towards it members. The introduction of the quasi-market in 1990s and consequent greater emphasis on decentralisation seriously undermined the FCC's power to influence. Nevertheless, the Government, which itself lacks the powers to directly influence the councils and the health care sector, still needed the FCC to create a dialogue with the county councils. Moreover, in the area of quality control, it provides funding to encourage, for example, evidence-based health care.

Clinical Guidelines and the Swedish Institute for Health Service Development. The Swedish Institute for Health Service Development (SPRI) was closed down in December 1999 following pressure from the Federation of County Councils. SPRI was established in 1968 and was formally and jointly controlled by the Ministry of Health and the Federation of County Councils. SPRI was established in 1968 and is formally and jointly controlled by the Ministry of Health and the Federation of County Councils. SPRI was established in 1968 and is formally and jointly controlled by the Ministry of Health and the Federation of County Councils. Initially its task was to provide the county councils with the appropriate methods for long-term planning of health care. By the 1980s the organisation had undergone major changes and it had become the main agency for the development of clinical guidelines within a broader remit of technology assessment and the 'efficacy, efficiency and humanitarian and social acceptability of medical procedures' (Jost 1992:82). SPRI and the Swedish Medical Research Council held a number of joint consensus conferences during that period providing, for example, clinical guidelines for care of myocardial infarction, diagnosis and treatment of cerebral haemorrhage and stroke. In 1988 SPRI undertook nine studies including a review of pre-operative routines, treatment of back pain and vascular surgery. While not without its supporters this work of SPRI was criticised for being too complex and standardised for day-to-day use in clinics (Jost 1992: 83).

Up until its demise SPRI acted, according to some commentators, as if it were an equal partner to its sponsors – the NBHW and the FCC (Garpenby 1999:410). This was viewed as inappropriate as both the two national bodies saw SPRI as a consultation bureau working for them at the national level, not as an autonomous organisation with its own agenda.

Involvement of professional bodies. In the early 1990s the Swedish medical profession was gently pressured by the state and county councils to participate in discussions around the quality of care. The SMA and SSM established a joint body for the purpose, the Medical Quality Council (MQC) (*Medicinska Kvalitetsrådet*). It has ten members with a chairperson nominated alternately by the SMA and SSM. This council has tended to concentrate on those quality issues that impact most directly on the medical profession including the development of a programme of medical audit. The profession, however, has been divided on how best to respond and has had difficulty agreeing on which audit methodology to adopt. This indecisiveness has limited the effectiveness of the council (Garpenby 1999:411). It is partly as a consequence of this both the NBHW and the FCC have been able to begin to carve out distinct roles for themselves during the 1990s. In line with their pre-existing roles the FCC has concentrated on political and administrative management at the local level while the NBHW has been focusing on working closely with the medical profession (SMA and SMM). The NBHW and FCC under the Dagmar agreement of 1996 did agree to the establishment of national guidelines (*Nationella riktlinjer*) for the purpose of ensuring common high-quality and evidence-based standards of care across the country. The responsibility rests with the NBHW in consultation with expert medical groups So far, however, only three guidelines have been published, on diabetes, stroke and on coronary care. There are three versions of each guideline, one for the profession, one for the county councils and one for patients (Garpenby 2002; see also European Observatory – Sweden 2001:54–6).

Quasi-markets and decentralisation in the organisation of health care delivery has had a particular set of implications for the Swedish medical profession. This can be seen particularly well in relation to issue of quality control. With central government being less directly involved in the delivery of care it has become relatively less reliant on the profession as compared to its relations with the county councils. This should not be overstated as the links between the state and the profession are particularly deep and long established. Nevertheless, concentration on quality control issues such as clinical guidelines and evidence-based medicine does begin to change the nature of that relationship. Rather than the state relying on the profession wholly for the quality of care the new relationship emphasises more the need for accountability and external monitoring. This encroaches on the autonomy of the profession although how far it may erode it remains to be seen.

Clinical governance: summary and comparisons

One must not assume that the introduction of clinical guidelines in The Netherlands has meant that these cover all or even most of the clinical work for they do not. Nor do hospital doctors routinely consult those that are in existence, for they do not. This is even truer of Sweden where there is little consensus as how best to introduce and utilise guidelines. It is probably safe to assert this to be the case wherever else they are introduced within Western medicine and this could lead one to the conclusion that their use will have a low impact on clinical practice (for example, Lomas, Anderson, and Domnick-Pierre 1989). This view would be mistaken for it is to misunderstand the nature of the changing relations between the medical profession and the state. The medical profession in The Netherlands adopted consensus clinical guidelines as a means of avoiding the inconvenience of routine medical audit within their own hospital departments. Yet while the specialists may not routinely access the guidelines for their routine clinical work they do actively engage in their construction. Moreover, as an organised profession they have been able to maintain the moral high ground in this issue, in contrast to its member's position over fee reductions and integration of their costs (fees) into the hospital budget.

The Netherlands hospital specialists are probably the most entrepreneurial working within the public sector in Europe while their counterparts in Sweden are the complete opposite. Their salaries have been integrated into hospital budgets since the 'Seven Crowns' reforms and they are seen and see themselves as integral components of the hospital management structure, more a civil servant than independent professionals. It is perhaps surprising then that they have had more difficulties in coming to terms with clinical guidelines. Whereas The Netherlands doctors will view these as providing a point of reference if needed Swedish doctors are far more conscious of the issue of accountability. For the Dutch hospital specialist clinical guidelines have been a professionally led activity and there is kudos in being involved in contributing to their development and little concern over policing their implementation for it is very largely a professional issue. By contrast, the Swedish system of quality control is not a professionally-led activity but is part of a broader politicised debate between national and local politicians reflecting the dynamic tensions of their competing interests. Yet it would be wrong to interpret this situation as one of proletarianisation (in terms of status) or de-skilling (in terms of work content) of hospital specialists. It is from within this network that the Swedish doctors most benefit.

Whereas the health care field in The Netherlands is constituted within a broader political culture of subsidiarity, that of Sweden is configured under the broad social democratic ethos of decentralisation. Both emphasises placing decision making as close to the activity as possible but each has very different outcomes. The Netherlands emphasise the corporate interests of the social actors in the 'middle field' (*Maatschappelijk middenveld*), including the profession and Church, while in Sweden it is the political interests of national and local politicians that predominantly determine the shape of the agenda on health care provision and to a considerable extent that of the medical profession too. However, whereas The Netherlands Government has been keen to curtail the independence of hospital specialists, the Swedish state would appear to have been reasonably content with the service provided by their elite and urbane medical profession over recent years.

The other major health profession is that of nursing. Nursing work borders that of doctors and has in recent times and in several countries given rise to professional disputes. This is far less apparent within The Netherlands and Sweden – although for rather different reasons – than in some of the other countries to be discussed. The discussion will concentrate on the professions' responses and adaptation to managed care and explore the distinction between 'nursing' and 'care', which would seem to have implications for the future of the profession.

Hospital nursing, professional aspirations and management

Hospital nursing in both The Netherlands and Sweden share much in common with all other Western European as well as North American and Australasian countries. There has also been over recent years a policy commitment to convergence within nursing provided by the European Community particularly in the areas of education, training and occupational structures (Salvage and Heijnen 1997). Despite the likelihood that the differences will narrow, however, there will continue to be systematic differences in nursing and its role and relations to the other actors (including patients) in the health care actor network or field.

The Netherlands and Sweden represent, respectively, examples of the Breadwinner (that is, Corporatist) and Universalist (Social Democratic) regimes (Lewis 1989, 1992). They therefore represent a case in which one would expect a clear distinction in terms of gender discrimination and in terms of whether women are assumed to be primarily 'wives and mothers' or 'workers' (see Chapter 2, Figure 2.2). The implications of this will be examined in relation to, first, the professional and union organisation of nursing; second, nurse specialisation and its implications for professionalisation; third, nurse involvement within management; and fourth, a discussion around the gendered nature of hospital routines.

The Netherlands

Nurses' professional and union organisations

In 1993 the National Centre for Nursing and Care (LCVV) was formed as a federation of professional nursing and care provider interests funded by the government (Oud 1997). In 1996 the influential General Assembly of Nursing and Allied Health Professional Groups (AVVV) joined the consortium. This body is itself a coalition of 43 professional organisations[12] in nursing and care, including probably the best known and possibly most influential among nurses, the National Nurses Association of The Netherlands (Nieuwe Unie - NU'91) as well as the more specialised Society of Nursing Scientists (VERVE). The Nieuwe Unie (NU'91) is also very much a nurses' trade union but then, in intent, so is the whole federation of LCVV with its mission: '[t]o contribute actively to improvement and strengthening the position of nurses and carers in The Netherlands...improving the quality of professional practice and of health care delivery [and] realising a higher social status for both professions' (LCVV 1997).

During the early and mid 1990s nurse education and training underwent a major reorganisation. Prior to then there were many courses available for nursing students and care workers but most were independent of each other and there was no overarching and consistent sets of standards or regulations (Netherlands 1997). Following a period of experimentation in 1991–95 a new modular qualifications structure has been produced which meets the relevant European directive.[13] The new system also meets the requirements of the Individual Health Care Professions Act (Wet BIG) that came into force at the same time (Oud 1997). The course leading to the qualification and title of 'registered nurse' lasts for four years (as it did before) and is at level 4 and 5 (the other levels relate to care workers and helpers). Entrance requirement is no more than 12 years of general education at 17 years old. Once the general programme has been completed students opt for one of four specialisations (Netherlands 1996):

1 patients with serious disorder (but not intensive care)
2 pregnant women, new mothers and children
3 patients with psychiatric illnesses and the mentally handicapped
4 chronically ill patients.

There are no separate post basic types of nursing but specialisation training is available, which is similar in Sweden (European Commission 2000) although, in marked contrast to their Swedish counterparts, The Netherlands' nurses are resistant to carrying out any work that can be seen as medical work. This they claim would undermine their nursing role and their caring relations with patients (Salvage and Heijnen 1997:56). This is also the position adopted by the German nurses (see Chapter 5) and it is the case in both countries that nurses' work autonomy is primarily sought outside of the hospitals and within the community. In part, the attraction of nursing work in the community is the same for nurses working within all types of European health care systems. There are, however, specific peculiarities of the corporate model of Continental Europe relating to the organisation and role of hospital doctoring that provide more disincentives to hospital nursing than elsewhere.

Nursing and hospital management

Nurses' involvement in hospital management is at the level of the ward or group of wards, commonly referred to as 'clusters'. They used to have representation on at the top of the hospital hierarchy but this has changed over recent years as was explained to me in March 1997 by a quality assurance manager of a general hospital: 'Formerly there was always nursing director, there was [a] medical a nursing and general or financial [director]...And the nursing director has gone...throughout the whole country...The director of patient care is almost [always] a doctor'. Much of the work developing and implementing 'clusters' has been carried out by the National Hospital Institute (NZI) and a leading figure within it described the rationale for the new arrangements, also in March 1997, in the following terms: 'you have the Director, you have the Medical Board, the medical staff, medical committee and they do things with each other and so on. [The] nurses are not on a high level... in the hierarchy. But...she knows the patient...[and] the process for the patient...The nurse play[s] a very important role, in that process'. He illustrated his argument with an example: 'The management team... for [a clinical] department, [consist of an] internal medicine doctor... and...the head nurse...on the same level'.

The comment is a little patronising, for while the new management arrangements may be more effective than previously at directly harnessing the expertise of nurses within the management system these reforms will have undermined any status and/or influence nurses had previously within the management structure of the hospital. It is hardly surprising then that Dutch nurses increasingly favour community nursing over hospital work for a career. The Institute for Care and Welfare (NIZW) carried out a review of alternative futures for the nursing profession in 1997 and reported that there is a strong trend towards home care nursing (Oud 1997:8–9). This is supported by a strong trend towards 'transmural nursing', as it is called, which focuses on the integration between nursing facilities in primary care and hospital in order to improve the quality and continuity of care, especially for chronically ill patients. This is a development particularly associated with The Netherlands Institute for Primary Health Care (NIVEL).

Gender implications

Around 95 per cent of all nurses are women (WHO 1994) while the majority of doctors are male[14] although very probably not to the extent that nursing is feminised. Nevertheless, the demise of the nursing director would seem to indicate a significant change in the gendered culture of the hospital. Previously, the doctors were organisationally separate, but assumed that they had overall control of nursing because they dictated the treatment of patients. Under the new arrangements the doctors will have more formal authority and responsibility in the management of the hospitals but nurses will now have the possibility of ensuring patient care as well as treatment is part of the process. Whether this happens is not clear, but the new arrangements make it possible. What is clear is that nurses prefer to pursue their professional careers in the community and away from medical involvement as far as possible. For them it is the 'caring' component of nursing that is the core to their professional activities. In Sweden the situation looks different although there are many areas of similarity too.

Sweden

Nurses' professional and union organisations

In Sweden the division between union and professional organisation is even more blurred than in The Netherlands – and between nursing and medical work. The Swedish Association of Health Professionals is the trade union and professional organisation for nurses and other health professionals (www.vardforbundet.se/english) There is, in addition, the smaller Swedish Association for Nurses. It is, however, the health professionals, organisation that is the key player as well as the national member of the International Council of Nurses (ICN), WHO and the Nordic Nurses' Joint Organisation (SSN). Unlike The

Netherlands and many other countries in Europe, Swedish nursing is fairly unitary. It also has a particularly practical approach to the profession.

The nurse education and training programme in Sweden is for three years' full-time study (compared to the four years in The Netherlands). It is divided between theoretical studies and clinical training. There is no standardised syllabus or curriculum, for this is the responsibility of the study programme committees locally. However, these must ensure their programmes comply with EC regulations relating to nurse education. Prior to 1977 nursing (*omvårdnad*) and nurse training was dominated by medical science and taught very much as a practical apprenticeship by 'observing and imitating' (Bentling 1992:169). Nurse education and training is now carried out within higher education and has claims to rest on a scientific basis, a claim that also involves a commitment to nursing research. This is one made across Europe and is partly mandated by the European Commission and partly reflects the continuing professionalising project of European nursing (Salvage and Heijnen 1997).

The Health and Medical Care Act (1982) laid down the expectations and demands society places on the trained nurse and marked the introduction of 'new nursing'. This was much influenced by the North American 'nursing theory'. It was characterised by a holistic approach to patient care and with an emphasis on a *capacity of feeling and empathy* as well as to be able to *document, develop and evaluate* their work (Bentling 1992). While the notion of 'emotional labour' or perhaps more accurately 'sentimental work' (Strauss *et al.* 1982, 1985) may have been relatively easy and comfortable to adapt to, for it codified important and previously implicit aspects of nursing work. Adapting to the nursing process more generally, however, was probably harder for as Sahlin-Andersson (1994:142, emphasis added) has commented:

> Previously, everything which the nurses documented, often only in the form of brief reminder notes, was thrown out once the patient had left the hospital. Only documentation produced by the doctors was saved. Now, the nurses' documentation is also saved in the patient record…Nonetheless, *oral communication* dominates the interaction among the nurses.

This is not peculiar to Sweden, the oral tradition is shared across Europe and it will be referred to again in relation to both French and

German nursing. It is embedded within the craft traditions of nursing: a 'mystery' learnt by watching and assisting. Nightingale had considerable influence in Sweden, through the work of the Red Cross in training nursing. This influence did much to systematise and organise nursing in a way that fitted nursing more effectively into the modern hospital but rather less in changing knowledge and skill base of nursing.

It was the reforms associated with the *Health and Medical Care Act* of the 1980s that professionalised nursing for the first time, at least, in the sense that it now had a recognisable and defined knowledge base. This development, much influenced by American nursing theory (for example, Benner 1984) and reflected elsewhere across Europe, underpinned the move of nurse education into the universities and the emergence of the 'academic professionalisers' (Melia 1987:163). In attempting to adapt American nursing theories to Swedish conditions nurse academics have been confronted with the ambivalence within Swedish nursing to 'scientific' nursing, particularly if it means leaving behind the practical nursing and patient care work. The dilemma for Swedish nursing has been how to avoid conflating the notions of 'nursing' and 'caring' (Bentling 1992).

Nurse specialists and specialisation

Swedish nursing has often appeared particularly advanced to outside observers at least in terms of the specialist nurses in radiology and anaesthetics. There appears to be no equivalent in The Netherlands (European Commission 2000). On completion of basic training the newly qualified nurse (*legitimerad sjuköterska*) may wish to specialise possibly in anaesthetics, radiology or intensive care. These post-basic nurse specialisations are not legally protected. With the exception of radiology nursing (*röntgensjukoterska*) all of the specialisation provide little in the way of autonomy from medical dominance and direction. The work of the radiology nurse, for instance, is driven by 'protocols'. A radiologist at a university hospital explained the process in June 1997 as follows: 'We have standard pre-actions [that is, 'protocols']...and... examinations where you have standard pre-actions, they are performed by a nurse...she takes all the pictures after a protocol. So, where the examination is not a part of...making the diagnosis...then it's done by a nurse'. By contrast, the anaesthetic nurse specialist does have some autonomy. Compare the following description provided by a specialist anaesthetist (June 1997) of anaesthetics nursing to the previous one (for radiology).

In Sweden [the anaesthetic nurses] are quite independent and well trained...right now when I am sitting talking to you, my case is [being] run by a nurse anaesthetist...I would say that our work [medical and nursing anaesthetists] is very much the same...our speciality is one of those where the doctors and the nurses...do, quite often, the same things...[although, as the doctor, we] do the critical points of the procedure.

The fact that there can be such a legitimate *laissez-faire* approach is interesting for what it tells us about clinical autonomy in Sweden – it appears to be very much craft based. But whereas the doctors gain from this autonomy the nurses have little incentive to specialise other than an intrinsic interest in the work. This is not an example of clinical specialisation leading to career progression; nor is there much career development to be found within nurse management. Instead the development of specialised nurses probably reflects the relatively low ratio of doctors to population throughout the last century further exacerbated during the country's period of rapid expansion of the 1950s and 1960s.

Nurse management

Swedish nursing has been relatively untouched by the hand of managerialism. To start with, it would be difficult for a nurse to hold a senior management position for there is commonly no nursing director (WHO 1996:31; European Observatory – Sweden 2001:47) and the doctors monopolise the departmental management (excepting the emergency department) for it is only from that professional group that the heads are selected. There is, as it where, an interprofessional paternalism underpinning the working relations between the two, nurses and doctors. At the ward level this relationship can probably reasonably summarised in the words of this doctor working on a neo-natal ward at the same hospital and at the same time as the specialists cited above: 'our nurses are working...independently...by themselves...We are very much dependent on their ability to observe and see when something is going not so good with a baby. And they are very good at that'. The point is not specific to babies either; similar comments were made in The Netherlands too. Any sense, however, that this implies equal but different status is unfounded. The nurses report to the doctors not the other way around.

Gendered hospital routines

In Sweden 92.4 per cent of the nursing workforce is female (WHO 2000c:16). To understand the implications for the day-to-day relations between the nurses and doctors it is useful to start with the daily hospital routine of the nurses' report.

> The day-nurses start work at 7 a.m. when all nurses meet in the nursing office. The office is located in the middle of the ward...The night-nurse reports to one of the day-nurses...[who] then reports to the rest...She reports on each patient...In its structure this report sounded...very much like daily small talk, like a conversation between members of a family (Sahlin-Andersson 1994:136)

Such reports are basic to hospital nursing work and are to be found in hospital work across Europe, although varying greatly in their length, detail and how people involved. The reports are intended to ensure a continuity of care and ensure the nurses on the new shift are aware of any problems their patients may present them with during their shift. Moreover, they are distinctly nurse events, totally independent from management and medicine. This contrasts with that other ubiquitous and better-known hospital routine, the ward round.

> Around nine o'clock the doctors' round usually begins. A couple of days a week the senior physician and professors attend these rounds. On other days the assistant physicians does it alone, generally with a group of medical students in attendance. First of all everyone attending the round sits down, and they discuss the patients one by one...It is the doctor...who leads the meeting. The doctors ask the nurse for some information, the nurse takes notes about the treatment and tests which the doctors have decided. These notes are signed by one of the doctors. (Sahlin-Andersson 1994:140)

Again, this description would be readily recognisable across virtually the whole of Europe (and much of the globe too). The point of citing Sahlin-Andersson's account, however, is to underline the way in which the ward routines ensure the (female) nurses are subordinated to the (male) doctors.

The consequence of nurses' modern history, to overgeneralise for the moment, has been to cast nurses into the role of the doctors' 'assistant' or 'technician'. The first role, often stereotyped as the 'handmaiden', is illustrated by the account of the medical round provided earlier. Sahlin-Andersson (1994:140) describes the situation in relation to Swedish nurses she studied in the following terms:

[There were] many occasions when it became obvious that nurses' work is seen in terms of adapting to others: to other people's work, to their demands and appointments, or to whatever might happen during the day. The nurses' work is *now-oriented* and characterised by constant adjustments of this kind. (*emphasis added*)

It is this 'time orientation', she argues, that reproduces the nurses' subordination to others. While Sahlin-Andersson is discussing Swedish nurses she might easily have been referring to The Netherlands and, to a greater or lesser degree, most of Continental and Southern Europe, as will become clear in the later chapters.

Dutch and Swedish nursing compared

Nursing in The Netherlands and Sweden would seem to be only relatively autonomous from medicine. The dominant profession would appear to be able to exercise its jurisdictional authority with little need to make explicit demands. In neither of these two countries is there any real evidence of the emergence of autonomous nurse practitioners. In Sweden the specialist nurses work directly with and for their medical colleagues, who have the ultimate clinical responsibility. In The Netherlands the nurses do not want to be specialists supplementing medicine, rather they prefer to work far away from their medical colleagues in the community. It is unlikely that the preference not to work within acute hospitals is because of any major conflict with medicine, rather it is because Dutch nurses define nursing as 'care' and caring fits particularly well in relation to looking after patients who are chronically ill and living at home. Interestingly the Swedish nurses too have a strong affiliation with the notion of 'care' and 'caring' that has made it hard for them to adopt whole-heartedly the new nursing models that were introduced from North America. The same also was the case with The Netherlands. There would seem to be a common European tradition reflecting originally religious vocationalism that has transmuted into the modern secular age. The difference between the two countries may be explainable in terms of the 'wives and mothers' versus 'women as worker' model discussed in Chapter 2. The Dutch nurses are both confronted by and imbued with the cultural values of the family central to the historical legacy of subsidiarity whereas their Swedish counterparts are not. They, instead, reflect the values of the social democratic ethos characterised in their craft of caring tradition. This gives rise to a (contradictory) response to the scientific or rationalist approach to nursing epitomised by the nursing process and new nursing.

Conclusions

Reviewing the evidence and discussion of this chapter it is clear that the 'quasi-market' and moves towards managed care impacted more on the hospital doctors than nurses. In the case of the Dutch specialists, attempts to contain costs at their direct expense was strongly opposed, partly because of the implications for their earnings, although the profession was riven with divisions on this issue. But it was also because of the perceived threat to their strongly and uniquely institutionalised professional autonomy emphasised by their separate organisational status within the hospitals. Swedish hospital doctors, by contrast, offered virtually no opposition to the reforms; they had long been an elite part of the bureaucracy. This difference also is also reflected in approach of the two countries professions, to quality assurance or control. Interestingly, there was little interprofessional connectedness on either of these issues. Nurses in The Netherlands appear to be content to exploit the opportunity that the rationalisation of hospitals and adoption of the 'transmural' policy to advance their interests in community nursing. In the case of the Swedish nursing, there appears to have been little direct impact at all.

In the next chapter the comparison is between two other countries, one of which was an early – and best known – adopter of quasi-markets in health care, namely Britain, and France which also introduced some aspects of the organisational innovations although always ensuring a strong Gallic flavour to them. The reason for their selection as comparative case studies, however, is that they represent key examples of unitary polities from within the Anglo-Saxon (neo-liberal) and corporatist traditions within Europe. Moreover, in terms of populations they are also much larger than Sweden and The Netherlands. The implications for the medical and nursing professions, in consequence, prove to be significantly different.

4
The United Kingdom and France: *Étatiste* Traditions

In both the United Kingdom (UK) and France the health care system has been highly centralised as was the case with the organisation of the public sector services in general, reflecting an underlying and parallel, *étatisme*. However, the form this has taken within each country has been rather different. UK represents the now classic 'Beveridge' model of a tax-funded state-directed national health system later adopted in Scandinavia and, more recently, Southern European countries, whereas the French health system is based on the 'Bismarckian' model and funded by sickness funds. As Esping-Anderson (1990:166–7) has pointed out, the social democratic potential of the Beveridge Plan was not ultimately realisable because the working-class basis for its success was not strong or cohesive enough to prevent the welfare regime becoming instead more of what will be referred here as a neo-liberal hybrid and the contributing 'strain' in the 'mix' is the social democratic. France too is something of a hybrid in that its health care system is corporatist (that is, Bismarckian) in its basic organisation and funding arrangements, but the French central state has ensured that it is the dominant organising force and not, in the case of health care, any of the health care actors and certainly not any of the health care professions. Unlike other corporatist regimes France has political culture that has actively rejected subsidiarity in favour of *étatisme*, legitimated by reference to Rousseau's principle of the 'general will' (*volonté général*). This is interpreted as the state's central responsibility is to interpret and represent everyone's interests, which is rather different from the notion of the 'middle field' (*Maatschappelijk middenveld*) which characterises the state in The Netherlands (see Chapter 3) and quite different from the German federal model (see Chapter 5). Pollitt and Bouckaert (2000:53) argue reasonably enough that, along with Germany, France is a key example of the *Rechtsstaat*, for the state is the central integrating force whose authority and legitimacy is based on its administrative legal system. However, France with its strongly centralised system of administration differs from Germany, where the constitutional law emphasises the decentralised powers of the *Länder*. France might be thought of as a 'pure' type of *Rechtsstaat* in that its administrative legitimacy and control are apparently not offset by the countervailing forces of municipal, occupational or religious communities of civil society (Esping-Anderson 1990:27). It is for all these reasons that the French case will be referred to here as 'quasi-corporatist'.

In terms of health care reforms and the impact of what has come to be known as New Public Management, the governments of the two countries adopted seemingly very different approaches. The UK administrations of the 1980s and 1990s were quick to embrace the principle of the quasi-market while the French Government of the time preferred to avoid it and sought instead to enlarge local political representation. Quasi-market thinking was not unknown in French health management circles, and the *hôpital-entreprise* (inspired by Reagonite and Thatcherite economic thinking) became the concept central to the hospital directors, discourse during the 1980s and a major plank of their union's (*Syndicat National des Cadres Hospitaliers* – SNCH) leadership's programme and promoted by a right-wing tendency within the SNCH (Griggs 1999:138–42). In the end, however, the *hôpital-entreprise* was no more than a populist rhetoric used as part of a strategy to seek greater autonomy for hospital directors.

Both the UK and French Governments during this period sought to contain costs in general and gain detailed cost control over hospitals, and despite very real differences between them there is evidence of a convergence of policy thinking even though this manifests itself in different policy practices reflecting their different institutionalised arrangements. This, it will be argued, is more a case of 'path dependency' challenged by crises or 'conjunctures', those 'fleeting comings together of a number of diverse elements into a new, single combination' (Wilsford 1994:257) rather than direct neo-institutional isomorphism even though the reforms have been rationalised by reference to a common rhetoric or philosophy (cf. Pollitt 2001). To revisit the Saltman (1997) argument presented in Chapter 2, there are three elements to convergence within health care systems: the social (values and norms, culture and history); the political; and the three elements of contemporary health care delivery: the configuration of scientific medicine, institutional management and provider payment mechanisms. In the cases of UK and France the health care systems have been reconfigured along similar lines but have remained rooted in their own distinctive institutional arrangements.

What did make the reforms possible in the case of these two countries was the ability of their unitary states to implement changes in the health care system even against the counterveiling powers of the medical professions (Light 1995). This has also had implications for the nursing professions of the two countries for, unlike many other European countries, the jurisdictional boundaries between the two professions have proven to be relatively permeable (although the emphasis should be on the 'relatively' rather than the 'permeable') with nursing being able to extend and possibly enhance jurisdiction and possibly its professional status too. The implications of the states' strategies for the medical and nursing professions in the two countries, however, have been rather different. The British doctors have long been strongly integrated and centralised through the BMA and the Royal Colleges (although this would appear to be changing) whereas the French medical societies have long been 'organisationally weak and ideologically divided' (Immergut 1992:85) as, too, have the medical unions. French nurses, too, are organisationally 'pluralistic' whereas it is only the Royal College of Nursing and a limited number of unions that represent UK nursing.

A particular theme to be explored within this chapter is that of 'governmentality' (Foucault 1979b, 1999) and the medicine. As in the other chapters, the issue of quality assurance is discussed, particularly in relation to medical work (for example, evidence-based medicine and clinical guidelines) and the issue of medical autonomy.[1] In the case of nursing, it is the interrelated set of issues of changing professional boundaries, nurse specialisation and professional autonomy that provides the key focus.

To summarise, this chapter discusses, in the following order: UK and French health systems, hospital organisation and the issue of managed care; hospital doctors, professional organisation and the quality of clinical care; nurse specialisation, extended roles and changing professional boundaries between nursing and medicine; and draws some conclusions.

Hospitals and health systems: UK and France

UK: From quasi-market to managed care

The UK in 1997 was spending 6.8 per cent of its GDP on health care compared with the European Union (EU) average of 8.5 per cent

(European Observatory – United Kingdom [UK] 1999:48), the only European countries to spend less are Ireland and Turkey. On the other hand, a higher proportion of the total spend is publicly financed – 83 per cent – than the average for other EU countries (75 per cent) (Wanless 2001:9). In 1996 there were 102,610 doctors employed within the service (European Observatory – UK 1999:81) of which 23,680 were hospital consultants and 34,360 junior doctors (that is, in training grades). In nursing for 1996/97 there were 425,700 whole-time equivalent nursing, midwifery and health visiting staff.[2] This translates as approximately 1.64 doctors per 1000 population (including general practice and hospital specialists) and 4.97 nurses (all nurses working in the community and hospitals) (WHO Statistics 2002). These figures compare with 3.03 doctors and 4.97 for nurses for France. A simple comparison highlights a distinctive characteristic of the UK health system: that there is a very low provision of doctors compared not only with France but to the rest of Europe too. To list the number of doctors per 1000 population for the other countries included here emphasises either just how poorly provided is the UK population or how overprovided is the rest of Europe: in The Netherlands the figure is 2.51, Poland is 2.96, in Sweden the figure is 3.11, Germany has 3.50, Greece is 3.92 and Italy a sizeable 5.54. One of the key outcomes of the low numbers of doctors in the UK has been to ensure the dominance of the medical profession within a state-run system of health care.

The introduction in 1911 by the Liberal government of Lloyd George of National Health Insurance was probably influenced more by Bismarck's Germany (Cartwright 1977) than market liberalism. It is very likely, as Keir Hardy and the Independent Labour Party at the time pointed out (Esping-Anderson 1990:64), that part of the policy's aim was to nurture splits within the working class as well as deal with the issue of the need for a reasonably health workforce, a key component of the Bismarckian strategy (see Chapter 5). Following the end of the 1939–45 War this element of health policy thinking was to change radically when the Beveridge reforms for the health service were introduced under a Labour administration. The intention of delivering a high-quality service 'free at point of delivery' for all was perhaps not the aim of all the stakeholders, but this is what the political rhetoric reflected (Klein 2001:20), and there was a consensus that it would contribute significantly to a post-war class settlement. Moreover, it was one in which organised labour won a considerable victory but institutionally it proved impossible for the movement to build on this in the same way that their counterparts in the Scandinavian countries were ultimately able to do (Esping-Anderson 1990:166–67). The dominance of the liberal values of individualism and the market alongside a continued patrician influence of traditional elite (aristocratic) families and coupled with the electoral victories of the Conservative Party during much of the following period ensured that the social democratic elements were never to be realised. Instead the National Health Service (NHS) became more a matter of providing value for money than high quality health care.

Organisationally the NHS's original structure was highly centralised and bureaucratic, with political accountability at the top but little effective operational control on the delivery of health care. Here everyone trusted the doctors and nurses to do their best. It was the medical profession that gained most from the NHS; in Eckstein's words (1958:3) the NHS was in effect 'a "doctor's measure" much more than a "patient's measure"'. In this position of medical dominance, the doctors were able to obstruct any initiatives from Government with which they disagreed, for while Parliament allocated resources it was the doctors who decided how most of the money was spent. This became a real problem during the 1970s when, similar to elsewhere in Europe, health spending rose exponentially as expensive high technology and new drugs became increasingly available. The demand was also linked to the other inflationary pressures including patients' greater expectations of the health care professionals and people's longevity – although in the latter case costs were also linked to 'low-tec' long-term care (Elston 1991:68; Ranade 1997:37–41; Wanless 2002, para 3, 19–26).

It was with the White Paper *Working for Patients* (Department of Health 1989) that quasi-market reforms were first officially discussed as a means of improving the efficiency of the NHS. The resulting organisational arrangements had many parallels with health maintenance organizations (HMO) found in the USA, which is hardly surprising given that the most influential adviser was their US advocate Enthoven (1985). This radical innovation followed on from the earlier Griffiths' Inquiry (1983) which had introduced a general management approach from the private sector to replace the consensus management based formally but ineffectively on interdisciplinary co-operation that existed at that time (Ranade 1997:116–17). The problem had been that the doctors had dominated local decision making with their own agenda. The Griffiths reforms, based on line-management accountability, were intended to directly challenge this medical hegemony with effective management control based on a comprehensive information system and resource management, including clinical budgeting (Cox 1991:103). The system of resource management was subsequently embodied in the White Paper *Working for Patients* (Department of Health 1989 para 2.15) which introduced the internal market into the NHS. The internal market is a mimic market (Klein 2001:155–6) which Bartlett and Le Grand (1993:33–4) conceptualised as a 'quasi-market' constructed to ensure competition based on good information and minimal transactional costs. Also, there is a need for the actors to be motivated and not simply rule following, although financial motivation should always be a driver for efficiency and not for any other reason. The health authorities were made responsible for identifying the health needs of the community and the purchasers of care from the hospitals, clinics and other health care providers of the services. Some general practitioners (GPs) – as fund holders – also became purchasers on behalf of their patients. Hospitals, in order to meet the requirements of the contracting arrangements, had to install quality assurance systems (Morgan and Potter 1995:167–8).

In the 1997 general election New Labour replaced the Conservatives in government. They replaced the language of the (quasi-)marketplace with a more managerialist one emphasising co-operation, 'high trust' and 'flatter' structures. All was set out in the White Paper *The New NHS: Modern – Dependable* (Secretary of State for Health 1999). Health authority purchasers where replaced by primary care groups (PCG), commissioning groups which were to be upgraded to autonomous primary care trusts (PCTs). In April 2001 the Health Secretary (Alan Milburn) launched another round of reforms. Health authorities were to be reduced in number and by 2004 two-thirds of the 99 health authorities were have been merged to form 30 'strategic' but less influential health authorities as most of their responsibilities have been devolved on to the primary care trusts in a policy referred to as 'shifting the balance of power' (Department of Health 2001a). This policy is unique within Europe in its intent to prioritise primary care and general practice over secondary care. In principle this relegates the acute hospital to a supportive role only and topples the hospital specialist from the apex of the health care system. This contrasts fundamentally with the approach in France. This apparent inversion of the NHS organisational structure is intended to enhance its responsiveness to patients' needs, and in effect introduces a notion of subsidiarity into the system with decisions being made at the local level. But care needs to be taken in assuming that because there are fewer centralised bureaucratic directives the central state is not exercising control. These reforms were centrally directed rather than a response to local demands.

These policy and organisational changes reflect a clear policy adoption of a particular kind of managed care within the UK that Light (1997:300) had discerned as taking place rather earlier. But with the formal dropping of the internal market rhetoric and replacing it with such terms as 'health improvement', the term 'managed care' has become even more applicable. It has been under the banner of health improvement programmes that primary care and acute trusts, along with, importantly, local authorities and particularly social services departments, have begun to attempt to work together in a systematic way. In Light's (2000:70) estimation 'clinically managed care is the most promising, evidence-based developments in health care' which is often not what is happening in the USA where the concept was born. In the UK context, just as with the introduction of the quasi-market, this too has been introduced in a 'Big Bang' (Klein 1995) although this time, as part of the Government's 'Third Way' thinking, it may be more 'commanding but not controlling' (Klein 2001:215) for despite the consumerist rhetoric this new NHS organisation still relies on professionals and managers making the decisions on the patients' behalf. The big hope, it appears, is that British patients will be happier with shorter waiting lists, comparable to the better-performing European countries, than with a free choice of doctor. This lack of choice of physician is in marked contrast to the French system – and that of other European countries – and this realisation (and the implications this might have on public opinion and voters) may well have been behind the Prime Minister's pledge in January 2000 to increase NHS spending from 3 per cent to 5 per cent per year in real terms to bring NHS spending up to the average for the European Union (Klein 2001:203). A rationale for the policy was provided by the Wanless Report (2001), which officially documented what had been known for a long time, that the NHS has been seriously underfunded for the quality of services it was intended to provide. In the longer term (that is, twenty years) the NHS budget should double in real terms, accounting for between 10.6 per cent and 12.5 per cent of GDP (*Guardian* 2002:17). Within this new system the hospitals have to be far more responsive to local health needs in providing specialist support service for the primary care trusts.

The other half of the managed care model is quality control. Before going on to discuss this in any detail it is necessary to present an account of the French public sector health service for comparison.

France: corporatist *étatisme*

Public health expenditure as a percentage of GDP for France was 9.9 per cent in 1997 (European Observatory – UK 1999:48).[3] France is middle ranking in terms of GNP per capita but third overall in health expenditure (de Kervasdoué *et al.* 1997:59), a contributing factor to the general satisfaction the French feel for their health care system (Mossialos 1997; *Guardian* 2000:3). Other factors include the range and choice of services even though this makes it one of the most complex in Europe (OECD 1992:45). The system is based on a hypothecated system of funding in which virtually everyone is covered by the statutory health insurance – sickness fund – (*Assurance-Maladie*) (Lancry and Sandier 1999:443). The largest scheme, *Regime General*, covers trade and industry sectors, which is 80 per cent of the population, and is financed by payroll contributions by employees and employers. The overall system is under state control and co-ordinated by the National Sickness Fund, *Caisse National d'Assurance Maladie des Travailleurs Salariés* (CNMATS), a public institution (de Pouvourville 1997:163). There are 22 regional sickness funds (*caisses régionale d'assurance maladie*) and approximately one hundred primary sickness funds (*caisses primaires d'assurance maladie*). These bodies are managed by autonomous boards of trustees comprising elected union representatives and appointed employer representatives.

The sickness funds cover only about 72 per cent of health expenditure, which is considerably less than the 85 per cent average for Europe generally (de Kervasdoué *et al.* 1997:65; de Pouvourville 1997:163). Typically the rate for reimbursement for inpatient care is around 92 per cent while for ambulatory (outpatient) it is only 70 per cent, and private (independent) practitioners' fees are reimbursed at around 74 per cent (de Kervasdoué *et al.* 1997:65–6). The shortfall, however, is typically not paid in cash by the patient but from private health insurance. France, unusually, has an extensive system of cost sharing which covers the public as well as the private sector in which 84 per cent of the population have private insurance (*mutualles*) (Kutzin 1998:92). The increase of co-payments was intended by Government to inhibit patient demand and assist in slowing down health care expenditure, an important goal given the need to contain public sector costs as part of the commitment to the Maarstricht criteria (Vail 1999:312).

French people have not responded to the rising cost of co-payments by reducing their demand for health services; instead, the citizens have taken out additional private health insurance. In terms of social solidarity (or inclusion) this reliance on private insurance disadvantages the disadvantaged, for it is the workers in small firms, the young and the unemployed who tend not to have private insurance (Kutzin 1998:103). There have been growing concerns about social exclusion as well as an awareness that the traditional approach is unhelpful as a policy instrument in tackling the problem (Bouget 1998:161). The problem has been that the corporatist arrangements for funding and delivering health care are socially deeply embedded and therefore not easily changed. The health reforms have been constrained by the pre-existing institutional arrangements. Wilsford (1994) has argued that this is best understood with reference to a path-dependency model. Thus attempts at trying to contain costs over the 1980s and 1990s have largely been in terms of adjusting the co-payments (*ticket moderateur*) component but in the mid 1990s attempts were made to bring about a radical change in the system. These were the Juppé reforms.

Juppé reforms

Alain Juppé, the Conservative prime minister of Chirac's 1995–97 presidency, introduced the reforms bearing his name on 15 November 1995. These were criticised for the autocratic manner in which they were introduced (Vail 1999) and proved to be extremely controversial but as, Lancry and Sandier (1999:463) have also commented, '[the] central proposals were nevertheless...being implemented' by the Socialist Government of Jospin from 1997. While the party ideology might differ the particular conjuncture of economic constraints and political pressures meant that whichever Government was in power would need to implement a raft of reforms aimed at controlling costs. As a long-term aim the Juppé Plan aimed to provide the means of clearing the debt of the *Sécurité Sociale* over a period of 13 years by means of an 'exceptional' income tax of 0.5 per cent. Specific to the health sector, Juppé proposals (Vail, 1999:322; Lancry and Sandier 1999:463–4) included the following:

- constitutional amendment giving Parliament powers to set annual spending limits
- reduced annual increase in hospitals' global budget
- increased patients' co-payment for hospital treatment from 50 to 70 francs
- an exceptional tax of 2.5 billion francs imposed on the pharmaceutical industry
- increased health contributions from retirees and unemployed.

The doctrinal principle, however, was not so much concerned with emphasising the need for financial prudence but rather the ideal of social security for all, which in the field of health care translates as a citizen-based 'right to the same benefits in kind for all' (Bouget 1998:162).

The *Assurance-Maladie* is now to provide universal coverage and replace the nineteen or so funds previously existing, coupled with a widening of sources of contribution to include general tax revenues as well as payroll contributions.

In order to introduce the reform the tried and tested strategy of divide and rule has been used against the medical profession with the medical generalists winning for themselves the agreement that patients will in future enrol with a single general practitioner (*médecin référent*) for treatment and referral to a specialist (Donozynski 1998:1545). The agreement is with the *Médecins Généralistes France* (MG France) and it would appear to be their reward for supporting the Juppé reforms, and crucially being the only signatory to an agreement which binds all the other medical syndicats (Lancry and Sandier 1999:468; Vail 1999:334). This concession, however, does not provide the *médecin référent* with the same gatekeeper powers as the general practitioner in the UK, for the reforms have not rescinded the patients' right to consult a specialist without a GP referral. It is unclear at present whether this arrangement will take root within the French system; 'medical nomadism', that is, consulting several physicians, is a right that French citizens have long valued (and which is shared with other countries that have or had corporatist traditions). Also, three other general practitioners unions as well as hospital specialists have objected strongly to the proposals. Nevertheless, the thrust of the reforms is clearly aimed at transforming a substantial number of office physicians into general practitioners as a means of controlling rising health expenditure, rationalising the division of labour between office physicians (located in the private sector) and (public sector) hospitals. Also recently and similar to the UK, attention has turned to the issue of quality assurance.

Hospital doctors, the medical profession and governmentality

Any account of health care reform gives the medical profession a key role, sometimes as the hero defending liberal principles but increasingly as the villain interested only in protecting its members' self-interest, 'a conspiracy against the laity' as G. B. Shaw put the point in an earlier time. The reality is a more complex one in which the hospital doctors' participation within the actor network of health care delivery has changed (translated) from one resembling medical dominance to something similar to managed care. Rather than being relied on to provide the direction and purpose for acute hospital services, British and French doctors have had to come to terms with the fact that that there has been a reconfiguration of the actor network and they are no longer able to exercise quite so much autonomy and influence as they once did. But, as suggested in Chapter 2, these changes need to be seen less as a process of proletarianisation and more a case of responsibilisation, that is to say, doctors in both countries will continue to enjoy autonomy and influence but possibly in a way more accountable and integrated within the hospital division of labour. First, a historical review of how the UK and French medical profession arrived at their relative status positions within their respective systems of health care delivery.

The UK health system and the medical profession: historical context

In the UK, and more particularly England, the Royal College of Physicians can trace their origins back to 1518 and the Royal College of Surgeons was established in 1797. Alongside these occupations worked the apothecaries – many surgeons also qualified as an apothecary. The profession's modern history, however, starts with the establishment of the Provincial Medical Surgical Association in 1832 (changing its name to the British Medical Association in 1855) and the passing of the Medical Registration Act in 1858 (Berlant 1975; Larkin 1983, 1995). Unlike France, however, the British state showed little interest in controlling medicine (Burrage, Jaurausch and Siegrist 1990) and this 'resulted in the hospitals falling under the control of the doctors' (Macdonald 1995:77–8). Wherever organised professionals[4] are employed there is a tension between professional principles and practice, and managerial concerns with efficiency. In UK NHS hospitals, prior to the Thatcherite reforms of the 1980s, these tensions were contained, according to Stephen Harrison (1999:51–2), by the acceptance of three principles.

1 All governments were committed to clinical autonomy and it was the role of management to support the doctors in providing medical care.
2 The formal organisation of the NHS was constructed to be consonant with clinical autonomy.
3 The practice of NHS management (that is, administration) was more a matter of diplomacy than management.

Despite the different organising principles between France and the UK the management–professional relationship was similar in both.

The medical dominance that is implicit in this arrangement was not the result of an indulgent state; rather the success of the profession lay, despite antagonisms, with its very collaboration with governments and in taking responsibility, on behalf of the state, the health care of the citizenry. Since the mid-nineteenth century the state in the UK has protected the interests of hospital doctors from the domination of insurance companies and friendly societies while at the same time insulating them from any patients' inability to pay for treatment. The National Health Insurance Act of 1911 can be viewed in this light as can the 1948 nationalisation of the health service. At the same time the British state was confronted with a medical profession that could exercise a suzerain power that at times appeared strong enough to counter any policy judged by the organised profession to be against their interests. The one challenge that finally came to seriously threaten the autonomy and dominance of the medical profession was exponentially escalating costs. These proved to be politically too great for any British government and in the changes that followed British hospital doctors were confronted with increasing demands for detailed accountability. The state–profession relations within France have followed a not dissimilar path – but embedded within its particular corporatist version of *étatisme*.

The French health system and the medical profession: historical context

Before the French Revolution (1789) medicine was organised on a corporate model much the same as elsewhere in Europe except the state was particularly powerful and was able to impose greater authority over the professions than was the case in UK (Abbott 1988:158). The *Société Royale de Médécine* was established 1778 (Foucault 1973:26–7) although its main purpose was to provide advice and research into public health matters not clinical medicine.

The French Revolution was a major disruption for the profession, as it was for most other aspects of society. The revolutionaries of 1789 believed in the Rousseauian principle of the 'social contract', which tolerated no interest groups. All universities and their medical schools were closed in 1791 and only reopened again in 1803 with the state once again directly controlling the organisation of the profession, including education, malpractice and professional confidentiality. The new arrangements, however, were 'operated along loosely democratic lines (Abbott 1988:158–9). Nevertheless, doctors were not allowed to organise independently of the state under the Chapelier Law, which banned all interest groups as being antithetical to the 'social contract' (Herzlich 1982:245).

It was not until 1892 that doctors finally obtained the law that made it possible for them to legitimately organise as a profession (Herzlich 1982:245). Only then were physicians able legally to unionise and to negotiate fees. It took another 35 years, until 1927, before doctors' professional autonomy became enshrined within a medical charter (Immergut 1992:94), one that reflected far more the interests of the medical elite than many medical practitioners who served the burgeoning industrial working classes. The four principles of *la médecine libérale* were and remain: (1) freedom of physician choice by the patient; (2) freedom of prescription by the physician; (3) fee-for-service payment; (4) direct payment by the patient to the physician for services rendered (Wilsford 1991:119). The charter did not lead to the cohesive integration of the medical profession. In contrast to the situation in the UK, in 1884 there were approximately one hundred and fifty departmental unions (*sydicats*) with a total of 3500 members (Wilsford 1991:105). In that same year 40 of the departmental unions joined together to form the USMF (*Union des Syndicats Médecaux Francais*). To get around the Chapelier Law, these organisations did not present themselves as interest groups but as organisations to defend the rights (*droits*) of physicians. It is perhaps because of this emphasis these departmental unions were characterised by particularism and factionalism, for it is easier to gain solidarity in support of concrete interests than it is abstract rights.

In the first decades of the twentieth century there were two issues that exacerbated the tendency towards fragmentation: the organisation of health care and the licensing of physicians. The first issue became particularly pressing in the period immediately following the 1914–18 European war when Alsace became again part of France (Wilsford 1991:106). Alsace was really an excuse for the debate, for it raised the possibility of greater independence from the state for the medical profession. If France had adopted the Alsace model, one based on the German federal corporate model (see Chapter 5) the doctors would enter into collective contracts with local sickness funds. The model appealed to the dominant doctors' union, the USMF, as well as to successive governments, but it contradicted the yet to be formally articulated, but strongly embedded within sections of the profession, principles of *la médecine libérale*. The argument split the profession for several years and, in 1926, a liberal rival to the USMF was established, the *Fédération des Sydicats Médicaux de France* (FSMF) and it was this union that drafted the medical charter (*la médecine libérale*) which was then adopted by the whole profession in 1927. The upshot was the reintegration of the profession with establishment of the *Conféderation des Sydicats Médicaux Français* (CSMF) in 1928 which combined elements of both factions (Immergut 1992:94). The second divisive issue concerned ethics and licensing. The tendency of the profession towards fragmentation plus the individualism embedded within of *la médecine libérale* limited the degree to which the profession was able organise and police any reliable system of self-regulation. It took another major European war (1939–45) to bring about changes. The *Ordre des Médecins* was set up by the Vichy government in 1940 (amended in 1945) to take on this role (Wilsford 1991:106). A model that was also adopted in The Netherlands at around the same time and similar to the arrangements in Italy and Greece also set up under authoritarian governments.

It was not until 1958 that the organisation of hospital medicine took on its present form. 'It is not an exaggeration to say that the Debré reforms are the most important attempt at change [of the French hospital system] which has been made since the...French Revolution (Jamous and Peloille 1970:120). The aim of the commission was to identify how best to reorganise hospital medicine and medical education along more rational and scientific lines. There were three central principles to the reforms:

1 *Better planning of the hospital system*: organised on a regional basis, with clear distinctions between types of hospitals. Government to control the growth of the independent hospital sector;
2 *To raise the status of public sector hospital specialists*: achieved by the creation of full-time senior salaried posts (*chef de service*) for doctors committed to high quality clinical work, teaching and medical research. Work in the independent (private) sector for public sector doctors to be prohibited.
3 *Appointments on the basis of merit*: based on competitive examinations and not on patronage, as was previously the case.

At the time the hospital elite and the urban practitioners strenuously opposed the reforms, for they had most to lose from their implementation (Immergut 1992:121–2). Younger doctors, on the other hand, saw the changes as a way of overcoming the rigid hierarchy of the hospital system and of improving their career opportunities. The provincial doctors were also sympathetic to the reforms because private practice in rural areas was not very lucrative and the reforms offered a secure income and career. The intensity of the conflicts within the profession, however, led to major splits and ultimately, in 1968, to the establishment of the *Fédération des Médecins de France* (FMF) which claimed to represent 13,000 doctors compared to 20–25,000 by the CSMF (ibid.: 273, fn. 102). However, the CSMF was able to re-establish its central negotiating role under the United Left Government of the time (Godt 1987:467). The impact of the Debré reforms on hospitals was slow to be felt but they have had a long lasting effect. Between 1965 and 1980 there was an expansion of 15,000 full-time posts (Immergut 1992:275, fn 114). The 1970 Hospital Law was based, in part, on the Committee's recommendation and, under the Socialist Government, private beds were eliminated from public hospitals in 1982.

The creation of the prestigious *chef de service* post as a lifetime and wholly autonomous appointment was intended to provide medical leadership, and in this the reforms were more or less successful. What was not realised sufficiently at the time were the cost implications of the policy, which contributed to an unsustainable escalation of health costs in the 1970s. But it also had the effect that growing numbers of young doctors actively chose salaried hospital appointment both for the career opportunities and the relative security it offered. It was not only, or even mostly, the *chefs de service* who added the inflationary pressure on health care spending in the 1970s, there were also other conjunctures that together had an even greater impact. First, there was the nationwide contract of the CSMF (Confederation of Medical Unions) with the national sickness fund (CNMATS) (Godt 1987:467), which drove health care costs up. Second, the then United Left Government found it politically impossible to reduce social and health benefits (to counter a threatened massive deficit) because of their reliance on the Socialist – Communist alliance for political support. Between these two forces the government found politically impossible to control and played an important part in the defeat of the United Left in 1978. The new right-wing government conceived a strategy involving the indirect control of the sickness funds and direct control of the hospitals. It included an increase in the patients' co-payments for prescription drugs and, even more fundamentally, in 1979 (Godt 1987:467–8) the Health Minister introduced the 'global envelope', which linked health expenditure directly to the country's GDP. The Government instructed the CNMATS (national sickness fund) to impose a new national contract with the doctors. Public sector hospitals at this time were spending 50 per cent of all health expenditure (ibid. 468): and part of the problem was commitment to *la médecine libérale* (see above) of the well-paid, salaried and autonomous *chef de services* and their imperviousness to appeals for cost restraint. New reforms were introduced in the early 1980s designed to bring costs under control in part by challenging these privileged 'mandarins' (ibid.:468–9), the most important being the 1983 law that introduced a prospective global budget which replaced the pre-existing per diem (day-rate) system[5] of payment with a set budget for each hospital paid in monthly installments (ibid.). The reform was not well received by the senior hospital specialists for it was seen as a managerialist strategy designed to make the *chefs de service* take budgetary responsibility for their departments (Griggs and Dent 1996:10) in a not dissimilar way to hospital consultants in the UK having to accept the same responsibility through the clinical directorates following the Griffiths Report. The reform was modified with the 1987 Hospital Law, which ended the lifetime tenure of the *chef de service* and from now on it was to be for five years, renewable by the Minister of Health. But to counterbalance this loss of tenure the 1987 Law reinstated the domain of the *chefs de service*, the clinical specialties (*service*), as the fundamental organisational unit and not management departments (Horellou-Lefarge, Joncour and Lararge 1990).

There then followed the crucial 1991 Hospital Law, which addressed the issue of health planning procedures and the limits to the regulated market for hospital services in France (Griggs and Radcliffe 1994:236). The basic framework was the health map (*carte sanitaire*), of 200 geographical health sectors, introduced twenty years earlier but extensively revised, which constituted the devolution of planning responsibility to the region (very much against the *étatiste* traditions of France). Together, the three Hospital Laws of 1983, 1987 and 1991 reshaped hospital provision from one that provided ample space for the professional dominance to one that demanded far more accountability from the senior doctors. The 1991 law to a large extent left the hospitals to decide their own internal organisation. It also introduced a specialty of nursing care (*service infirmier*) providing, for the first time, a forum for nursing policy across the hospital (Griggs and Dent 1996:12). The general thrust of the 1991 law has been towards greater decentralisation of the public sector hospital system. While it would be inaccurate to refer to these changes as marking the introduction of a quasi-market as in UK, there are parallels.

UK and French hospital doctors and governmentality

It might be argued, as Godt (1987:477–8) did in the 1980s, that the changes within the British and French health care system, particularly in relation to cost controls, weakened the medical profession vis-à-vis government. 'The professional power of the physicians has been marshalled in one way or another to accept…reforms, despite initial resistance. Although this result does not necessarily mean the doctors have been defeated' (Godt 1987:477). This notion of professions having to comply to state demands in order to avoid being defeated reflects some parallels with governmentality (see Chapter 2), for as Johnson (1995:20) has argued, as government objectives alter, transforming the boundaries of politics, so too do professional jurisdictions and the established powers and functions of the state'. The point is central to Foucault's view of governmentality.

Governmentality would seem to be particularly appropriate to contemporary French medical profession given the context of strong state and Rousseauian political philosophy (that is, the state encapsulates the will of the people). In this context the role of the medical profession appears to be more Gramscian than Durkheimian. In other words, the medical profession are equivalent to 'organic intellectuals' (Gramsci 1971) and thereby part of the state apparatus. At the same time the professions – and particularly doctors – are far from being 'docile bodies'. In Anglo-Saxon countries the issue of autonomy historically relates directly to the notion of a profession's collective identity via the strongly independent and influential role of the medical colleges, societies and associations, for example, Royal Colleges and the British Medical Association (BMA) in the UK. In France, by contrast, the medical associations (*Sociétés Savantes Savants*) and the medical trade unions are much more fragmented. Initiatives always come from the state, yet the state is not viewed as a restriction on the profession, for if the profession is well enough connected and organised government regulations relating to them will reflect their interests. One area in which state – profession relations are particularly central is that which in the UK is known as clinical governance, which covers the issue of quality assurance, medical and clinical audit as well as guidelines, evidence-based medicine and practice. Clinical governance is, in part, an organisational arrangement for attempting to ensure the accountability of the physician to the hospital as well as promoting 'best practice'. As explained in Chapter 2 this is, or has been, a contested terrain, and even where systems are in place their role may be as much 'myth and ceremony' (Meyer and Rowan 1991) to underpin legitimacy as they are systems of quality control. This may be an overly cynical view.

Quality assurance and clinical governance

Quality assurance systems can be understood as a latter-day version of the 'panoptic gaze' (Foucault 1979a) and it is this aspect of quality control systems that has led medical professions to be very wary of them. In UK they were introduced first within the hospital sector and have been more recently demanded of general practitioners too, whereas in France the direction was the other way around. The general argument presented will be that we have seen a shift of emphasis from a professional (institutional) accountability to a managerial (organisational) accountability, which I will label Governance I and Governance II in order to emphasise the continuities between the two as well as the differences.

Clinical governance and British medicine

For over thirty years, attempts have been made by British governments to get the medical profession to implement systems of accountability. The General Medical Council (GMC) – the doctors' professional 'watchdog' – had (and has) responsibility for ensuring that 'bad' doctors are brought to account, but the system has proven to be clumsy and inept and has lost much credibility even among the profession itself. Currently (2003) the Government is introducing an 'overarching council' that will oversee the work of the eight statutory regulators including the GMC (Dewar and Finlayson 2002). For medicine, this is seen as necessary in order to regain public confidence following recent scandals including that of children's heart surgery at the Bristol Royal Infirmary (Kennedy Report 2001). While the proposed change is an important one it will not impinge directly on doctors' clinic work. Here other controlling mechanisms have been tried.

Governance I. Accountability and quality assurance

Quality assurance in relation to health care delivery is a term that can cover any systematic activity designed to maintain or improve patient care and may be controlled or driven by management or profession. Figure 4.1 illustrates the situation within the UK. I am using the appellation 'Governance I' to identify the first generation of quality assurance methods which were innovations introduced within the profession and are intended to be self-managed by the profession (even if also promulgated by the state). British medicine was a relatively early adopter of medical audit, a key example of a professionally driven system for doctors (Dent 1993). Clinical guidelines (see Figure 4.1) are based on the principles of prospective audit. In The Netherlands (see Chapter 3), for instance, the hospital specialists favoured consensus guidelines as an alternative to medical audit meetings. In the UK, however, doctors' inertia in relation to medical audit led to the emphasis switching to a multi-professional approach (NHS Management

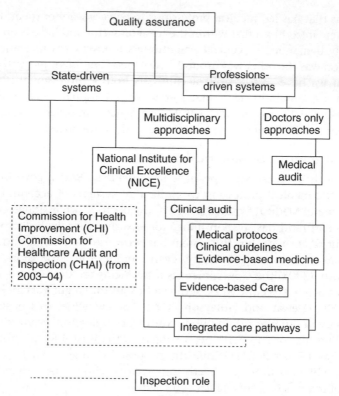

Figure 4.1 Quality assurance systems for hospital medicine in the UK (*simplified*)

Executive 1994; Department of Health 1994), which effectively meant a nurse-led approach. Within the medical profession the realisation that their clinical autonomy might well be under threat led to an acceptance, if not embracement, of evidence-based medicine (EBM), for this approach asserts the centrality of scientific medicine (Sackett *et al.* 1996; Sackett and Wennberg 1997; Harrison and McDonald 2003).

Governance II: Governance as 'responsibilisation'

Integrated care pathways, the next stage on from evidence-based medicine and care, cross the 'Governance I/II' border. They probably started out as instruments of managed care in the USA and are built up from the knitting together of protocols and guidelines of the different professional groups involved along a common time-line in order to deliver effective and efficient care. In principle this may well be true although in practice the situation is far more complex, for it is reasonably well documented that doctors tend to use guidelines as just that – suggestions to be followed if thought appropriate whereas, nurses tend to view them as rules to be obeyed (Parker and Lawton 2000). In addition, there would appear to be no clear consensus as to how detailed pathways need be or how closely they need to be followed. It is not entirely clear when and whether they are explicit instructions or helpful exemplars. Nevertheless, they do constitute a crucial component of the means for delivering the British Government's agenda for high-quality and efficient health care delivery.

An important part of the New Labour agenda – in addition to their claims to reject the 'quasi-market' approach – is a commitment to subsidiarity (even if this term is not in common usage), in terms of delegating authority and autonomy to hospital and primary care trusts. The powers of these autonomous organisations, however, are contained within a wider regulatory framework that includes the following agencies:

1 *National Institute of Clinical Excellence (NICE)*. Has the responsibility for evaluating drugs and therapies and to give authoritative advice to all health professionals. In addition to producing clinical guidelines the agency is also concerned with reducing waiting times, and developing new services.
2 *National Service Frameworks (NSF)*. Set standards for certain conditions for which the provision and quality of care is patchy across the country. These include heart diseases, mental health problems and diabetes One key outcome is likely to be locally negotiated care pathways based on national criteria.

To ensure 1 and 2 are acted upon the following agency has been established:

3 *Commission for Health Improvement (CHI)*. An independent body, to be replaced in 2003–04 by the Commission for Healthcare Audit and Inspection (CHAI) (Cabinet Office/Department of Health 2002). Both CHI and CHAI provide an independent inspectorate of all NHS hospitals, community and primary care services. The performance measures that underlie this process have been developed by the Department of Health, working with NICE, Audit Commission and, importantly, the Royal Colleges of the medical profession.

This regulatory framework involves not just the medical profession, but all the other health professions too, as well as the managers. There are other agencies involved but peripheral to the account here (see Walshe 2002). Similar developments are discernable within the French health systems too.

Quality of care and French medicine

There is probably greater ambivalence within the French medical profession over the issue of quality assurance than among their British counterparts. Until relatively recently doctors were only accountable to themselves for the efficiency and quality of care. It was part of *la médecine libérale*. Sickness funds have the responsibility to review a sample of medical records regularly to ensure adequate care has been provided but these audits do not question clinical judgements (de Pouvourville 1997:167); the sickness funds are more concerned with financial consequences. As the pressures for cost containment intensified during the 1980s so did concerns relating to the quality of care and sickness funds intensify their local audits. It would appear that the doctors in the independent sector were providing more services than were medically required in order to compensate the new lower fee schedule. The 1992 report of the Chief Medical Advisor of the National Sickness Fund brought the whole issue to a head referring to the 'waste, abuse and deception' of medical practice within the sector (ibid:168). The medical profession in the independent sector reacted to the pressures from the sickness funds and government by arguing, in a similar vein to the hospital specialists in the UK for the introduction of rational scientific criteria. They wanted the introduction of medical-ized control rather than accounting control (ibid:168). This was the task that was taken on by the *Agence Nationale Pour le Développemment de l'Evaluation Médicale* (ANDEM) created in 1990 not only for this purpose but, like NICE in the UK, to assess and advise on medical innovations, new drugs and safety issues. ANDEM was the outcome of a government report (Armongathe 1989) and established to encourage the adoption of EBM and develop medical technology assessment methodologies. In 1992 a law was passed that introduced legally binding clinical guidelines, *Références Médicales Opposables* (RMOs). These would be progressively introduced but initially at least would apply primarily to the independent sector and non-compliance would incur financial penalties. Twenty-four national guidelines were introduced in 1994, which together were predicted to save the National Sickness Fund 10.7 billion francs. The expectation was that eventually there will be more than 200 such guidelines (de Kervasdoué *et al.* 1997:71). The system is policed by the local medical joint committees, which include representatives of the professional associations and the sickness fund. According to de Kervasdoué *et al.*, even though RMO guidelines claim to be scientifically based and are approved by experts of the doctors' unions and ANDEM, they lack credibility within the medical profession because they are seen more as instruments for cost containment than quality promotion.

Pressure for the adoption of quality assurance systems within the hospital sector came from growing concerns over safety and effectiveness as much as costs. A particular impetus was the news story of the late 1980s that reported over half of the country's 2500 haemophiliacs had been infected with HIV from blood transfusions. The fatalities of this awful accident accounted for 56 per cent of all such deaths in Europe (*Guardian* 1999). There were also growing concerns within the state administration over the effectiveness of care and treatment, for example, in maternity units and emergency rooms, which led to the adoption of a policy of concentrating medical and nursing services in specialist centres to ensure the doctors dealt with sufficient complex cases to maintain their expertise (de Pouvourville 1997:168).

Under the 1991 hospital law, the assessment of the quality of care became a mandatory objective and gave rise to the creation of the *Programme Hospitalier de Recherché Clinique* (PHRC) designed to encourage clinical research by hospital-based doctors. In 1994, it also saw the introduction of the *Programme Assurance Qualité* (PAQ), although this was more concerned with total quality management principles than directly with clinical practice. More recently, the issue of accreditation has come on to the agenda and in 1998 ANDEM was expanded and has changed its name to ANAES (*Agence Nationale d'Accreditation et d'Evaluation*) and is now responsible for accreditation across the public and independent sectors (de Pouvourville 1998). The process, which is mandatory, was implemented in 1999. The body includes representatives from the medical profession and the sickness funds and is funded by Government and the national sickness fund.

Quality assurance comparisons: UK and France

Despite similarities between the UK and France in relation to the issue of quality assurance there is a key difference too. The similarities are between the NICE and the original ANDEM and there is also comparability between the role of ANAES as the accreditation agency in France and CHI as the hospital inspectorate in the UK. The key difference is that in France clinical guidelines in the form of RMOs are legally enforceable, which is not the case in the UK where compliance is scrutinised by CHI (Commission for Health Improvement) and exhorted by government and professional bodies (for example, Royal Colleges). The outcome is probably very similar and it is unlikely that hospital doctors (and other health professionals) in either country can avoid familiarity with clinical guidelines. The system of regulation and monitoring is formally external to the organised profession and can be viewed as enhancing the 'responsibilisation' of the profession, to borrow Fournier's (1999) useful term. No longer is it sufficient for the medical profession to claim to audit their own activities because they know best how to deliver good medicine safely now it has to be shown increasingly to be evidence-based and authorised by the appropriate body. This marks the boundary between 'Governance I' and 'Governance II'. Nevertheless, it is also important to note that in both countries the medical profession significantly influences these very external regulations. It is leading members of the profession who have a major input in establishing the rules and, in the UK, the Royal Colleges and medical researchers provide the evidence base for new medicines and shape the care pathways. All of these changes indicate a reconfiguration in the relation between the professional jurisdiction of the medical profession and the powers and functions of the British state and, in the process, of governmentality too (see Johnson 1995:20, quoted above). Another dimension to the professional jurisdiction of the medical professions of the two countries relates to the permeability of the occupational boundary between medicine and nursing.

Hospital nurses: extended roles and professional boundaries

Like medicine, hospital nursing in the UK and France also share certain similarities despite being of different welfare regimes. This has less to do with isomorphic convergence (DiMaggio and Powell 1991) and more to do with the dynamics of governmentality within strong unitary states, even though European Commission regulations relating to nursing education, training and labour market mobility are an example of a mix of coercive and normative isomorphism in that member states have to comply to the regulations but these have been established with a substantial input from the professional bodies (for example, Stallknecht 1992). For a start, compared to nursing across Continental Europe the professions within France and UK would appear to have achieved much in the way of professional autonomy and status, although this is not the same as stating that the organised professions in the two countries have achieved all that they would wish. Nevertheless, this relative success of nursing in these two countries stems from the Faustian pacts they have entered into with the state, rather than their effectiveness at gaining autonomy from the state (and medicine). This is different, too, from the situation in Scandinavia (as the discussion of the Swedish case in Chapter 2 demonstrated), for the work-based professional autonomy and expertise there is more rooted in the doctor – nurse division of labour and the craft traditions of nursing. Also, and related to this state – profession compact, nursing in both countries plays a strategic role in the co-ordination of the hospital division of labour, especially in relation to the allied health professions. Senior hospital nurses in both countries have increasingly taken over the responsibility of the co-ordination the allied health professions (for example, physiotherapists, dieticians etc) around the patient and this is reflected in their senior management role within hospitals in both France and the UK.

The French and UK represent, respectively, examples of the 'Breadwinner' (that is, corporatist) and a variant of the 'Minimalist' (liberal) regimes (see Chapter 2). One would therefore expect a clear distinction between the two countries in terms of gender discrimination although in practice the distinction is rather less clear, for the étatisme of France has more in common with the UK, particularly in relation to nurse professionalisation, than it does to other corporate states. Since the French Revolution the unitary (*étatiste*) French state has, been keen to counter the subsidiarity and familialism that has shaped gender relations more elsewhere in continental and Southern Europe, which in turn has shaped the profession's weaker jurisdictions in those countries. In the UK, governments have shown a willingness to offer nurses opportunities to extend there work into more specialist areas, in part as a strategy of reconfiguring the health care division of labour in order to deliver care more efficiently and effectively. This has meant routine nursing care increasingly being taken over by health care assistants and routine medical procedures being taken over by nurses. In this process the language of professionalisation provides a useful rhetoric.

This comparison of French and UK nursing is organised as follows: (1) history and professional organisation of nursing; (2) hospital nursing and gender (3) nurse specialisation and professionalisation; (4) nurse and hospital management.

History and professional organisation of nursing

Despite the different history and background there are considerable similarities between the nursing professions in France and UK. There are, as must be expected, a number of distinctive differences too. For instance, there is a Catholic tradition within France which is reflected even more strongly in other countries of mainland Europe but not shared by the UK. On the other hand, Nightingale's regime for nursing and nurse training was influenced by the work of Anglican nursing sisterhoods (Cartwright 1977:155). There were other important contributors to modern nursing in the UK too including Elizabeth Fry, Louisa Twinning and Sister Dora (Williams 1980:44). The institutional context of nursing within the two countries had also become secularised from a relatively early date (that is, not overtly ecclesiastical). French hospitals passed into municipal control in the seventeenth century (ibid.:36) while the voluntary hospitals, unsupported by 'Church, State or ratepayers' were well established in the UK by the eighteenth century (ibid.).

It is, of course, Florence Nightingale who is cited by all as the founder of modern nursing, not only in the UK but also across Europe too, often through the medium of the Red Cross as in the case of Sweden and Greece. But in most European countries, including France, Nightingale became a touchstone for local initiatives and programmes. In France secular nursing was slow to develop and it was not until 1902 was the role of the nurse in its modern form defined legally (crucial within the French tradition) and the schools of nursing received their formal assent (Quinn and Russell 1993:77–8). It was not until 1922, however, that the first nursing qualification (*Brevet de Capacité Professionel*) was legally recognised. It was also about this time, in 1919, that the Nurse Registration Act went on the UK statute book (Witz 1992:162–3), which in many ways paralleled the French case. In France, as explained in relation to the medical profession, it is not autonomy from the state that a profession sought but regulations by the state that embodied their rights to autonomy. This is similar to Larson's (1977) Weberian concept of a heterogenous profession, as opposed to the autonomous variety, which the UK (but not the French) medical profession represented. The first derived status and rights from within the state (and this applied equally to medicine and nursing within France) while the latter functioned more as a fiefdom and was able to function largely autonomous from the state. The Nurses Regulation Act (1919) in many ways reflected better the model of state – profession relations and suited the mix of legitimacy and accountability required by a modern democratic but unitary state relying on expert labour (for example, profession) for health or welfare services to its citizens. In those terms the Medical Registration Act (1858) was historically an anomaly, which no other European state cared to emulate. As a consequence, discussions about the limitations of the Nurses Registration Act (1919) may well be misplaced, for they have taken the nineteenth-century medical model of practitioner autonomy as the ideal. In practice, UK nursing has been fragmented less by the failure of the Registration Act and more because of external reasons impinging upon its members ability to act cohesively in establishing a strong professional identity and underpinning organisations. There are similarities here with the French situation too. First, the nursing jurisdiction has been dominated by medicine; second, nursing is predominantly a female gendered occupation; and, third, it was not in the interest of the state to facilitate a fully autonomous nursing profession (the medical profession was sufficient for purposes of delivering public sector health services). The first two characteristics are common to the nursing profession across Europe, the third is not in the sense that the French and UK central states have had the power and authority to act in a way others have not, for self-evidently they are not federally constituted, nor do they suffer the lack of authority of the Southern European states or the challenges of the East European states (see Chapters 5 and 6). One of the implications of this is that the French and UK states have real power to influence, amend or change the jurisdictional boundaries between nursing and medicine which from time to time they have exercised. This is in part because nursing and medicine is drawn right into the centre of government.

Nursing within the UK is represented at the level of the Department of Health with a chief nursing officer for each of the four countries (England, Wales, Scotland and Northern Ireland). The French profession is not, but has instead technical advisers responsible for advice, representation and assistance (WHO 2000a, 2000b, para. 3.4.1). They amount to much the same thing in terms of function and influence but do reflect the difference between the two professional models. In both cases but via different routes advice and influence is channelled between the institutions where nursing and nursing education and training takes place and the government ministry. The real difference between the two systems is the fragmentation of the French nursing professions and union representation compared to the UK.

For reasons similar to medicine, French nursing is represented by a large number of organisations. The figure varies between 60 (WHO 2000a:19) and more than 120 (Paquier 1993:81). The main organisation for public sector hospital nurses is ANFIIDE (*Association Française des*

Infirmiéres Diplômés et Élèves) established 1924 (Paquier 1993:81). In addition to the professional associations and nursing unions the larger general trades union have sections for health workers, including nurses. The main examples here would be the CGT-FO (*Confédération générale du travail-Force ouvrière*) (historically the communist union for manual workers) and CFDT (*Confédération Français démocratique du travail*) (historically a Catholic union for white-collar workers, although now more a white-collar union than a Catholic one). Professional activity is largely related to nurse education and training while activism in relation to nursing work is much more directed through union channels.

In contrast to France, the UK nurses are basically, divided between two organisations: Royal College of Nursing (RCN) and UNISON. The largest nursing organisation in the UK in terms of membership is the RCN. There were 425,700 (whole-time equivalent) nurses, midwifes and health visitors in 1996/97 (WHO 2000, para. 3.2) of which over 300,000 were members of the RCN. The RCN functions as a professional association, trade union and as an institute of advanced nursing. There is also the much smaller Joint Committee for Professional Nursing, Midwifery and Health Visiting Association. The main union representing nurses is Unison (formed from an amalgamation of the three main public sector unions in 1993), which represents not only or mainly nurses but many workers from the public sector in health, education and local government. MSF (Manufacturing, Science and Finance) also represent nurses (along with craft, technical, and some medical staff) within the NHS (European Observatory – UK 1999:23). As in the case of medicine, pay has been determined through the mechanism of a pay review body (PRB) rather than direct management – union negations. This body invites submissions from all parties then makes recommendations to government as to pay and conditions of service. The introduction of autonomous hospital trusts (and other varieties in the community, including primary care) has not changed the system of centralised pay review in favour of local negotiations.

Hospital nursing and the gender mix

The title of nurse (*infirmier*) within France is legally protected and subject to extensive regulation. Nurses are registered with the Board of Health and Social Affairs of the department in which they wish to work and will have completed a three-year diploma of state (DGS/DHOS 2002a). Within the UK all nurses, having completed a three-year diploma course, have to be registered with the Nursing and Midwifery Council (NMC) (since April 2002) a corporate body that has replaced the UKCC (UK Central Council for Nursing, Midwifery and Health Visiting) originally set up in 1983. The new body would appear not to mark a radical departure of its predecessor, but more of a fine-tuning reorganisation in order to fit better the Government's view that the professions within the NHS need to have greater lay representation and to be more transparent to public and government scrutiny (Department of Health 2001b: para. 2.3). This is all part of a 'responsibilisation' strategy (Fournier 1999) on part of the state but one that is intended to bite more deeply into medical autonomy than that of nursing. Its key responsibilities, in addition to maintaining the nurses, midwives and health visitors register, are listed as follows: setting and improving standards; advisory; dealing with misconduct and professional incompetence; quality assurance (O'Dowd 2002:11). There is no law listing what work a nurse may or may not undertake. Under the professional code of conduct a nurse is required to work within her level of competence. This means that the boundaries of nursing work can change relatively easily if the change is viewed as improving care in some way. Within the NHS boundary changes have been around the rise of the specialist nurses.

There are currently around 418,000 practicing nurses in France the majority of whom are employed in the public sector with only 14.2 per cent are employed within the private (*libéral*) sector. French nursing has one of the highest proportions of male nurses employed in Europe at 13 per cent (DGS/DHOS 2002a) although Italy, Switzerland and Spain are significantly higher (Salvage and Heijnen 1997:74, Fig. 5). The figure for the UK is a little less at 10 per cent (European Observatory-UK 1999:76). Clearly the profession in both countries and across Europe generally remains overwhelmingly female.

Unlike other corporatist regimes within Europe, there is little or no room within the French étatist system for family or religious affiliations to impinge directly on the gendered construction of nursing. On the other hand, the very concept of profession is itself a masculine one and, as Davies (1995:60–61) has pointed out, professional autonomy is masculine, rational and based on short client-encounters supported by extensive bureaucratic records and dependent on adjunct professionals and technicians to provide necessary support. This would appear to be essentially the same across Europe despite other differences as to the role of the state and universities (see Burrage, Jaurausch and Siegrist 1990). Nevertheless, in both French and UK nurses appear to remain actively committed to the Sisyphean project of professionalisation. A relatively recent advance in France, in this connection, has been the official recognition of an independent domain of nursing work. According to the WHO (2000a:12) document, the role of the general nurse is officially based, following the decree of 15 March 1993, on a 'bifocal model':

- independent care relating to the maintenance of life and compensation of lost independent function of the patient
- dependent role, which is under the direction of a doctor;

To which is added a third element:

- interdependent role, which is unspecified.

This is implicitly the same in the UK although this has not been spelt out, although developments of nurse specialists or practitioners imply just this kind of tripartite role (WHO 2000b: para. 3.3.8) – unless one is to assume unrealistically that nurses will take over all the activities carried out by doctors. In the French case, the clarification of the division of responsibilities, at least in a general sense, between nursing and medicine contrasts to the pre-existing model that emphasised the dependency relation of nurses on medicine for direction. There had been much unrest within the profession in the last decades of the twentieth century and in October 1988 there was a particularly crucial strike (Paquier 1993:84), which lasted nearly four weeks. In addition to demands for higher salaries, improved working conditions and a review of the career structure, the strikers demanded 'a recognition of the nurse's contribution to health' (ibid.). It is this latter demand that is contained within the 1993 reform, which identified for the first time the 'independent role of the nurse' although given the relatively high level of medical staffing (3.03 per 1000 population) compared to the figure for the UK (16.4) (WHO Statistics 2002) there is less room for the French nursing profession to establish the degree of 'independent practice' as has developed in the UK and other Anglo-Saxon countries, although, in the case of France, the situation is far less constrained than in other 'corporatist' European countries.

Specialisation and professionalisation

There has been a long tradition of hospital specialisation as theatre nurse (*infirmierde bloc opératoire*), anaesthetic nurse (*infirmier anesthésiste*) and paediatric nurse (*puéricultrice*), a more recent development of establishing nurse consultants within clinical specialties. The latter have much in common with similar developments in the UK (see below) while the earlier forms of nurse specialisation appear to be of more pragmatic origin sharing, unusually perhaps, some parallels with Sweden. Anaesthetics training for nurses was first introduced in 1947 in Paris (Maroudy 1996:15) and gained legal recognition in 1960. Even so, many anaesthetic nurses in this earlier period and right up to the late 1970s would work unsupervised because of the lack of anaestheticists. Some elements within the medical profession wanted to abolish anaesthetic nurses but due to the lack of realistic alternatives the solution to improving the quality and safety of anaesthesia service was the upgrading in 1988 from a certificate to a diploma in anaesthetic nursing. Currently there are 6044 such nurses and they include the highest proportion of male nurses (27 per cent) (DGS/DHOS 2002b). The responsibilities of the operating theatre nurses would appear to be comparable to those of their UK counterparts although within the NHS there does not appear to be a specific nurse specialism as in France. The core responsibilities here are the maintenance and sterilization of operation theatre equipment and supplies. The gender mix here is more in line with nursing generally, with only 12 per cent being male (DGS/DHOS 2002c). Paediatric nursing only is 99 per cent female in composition and requires less training than the other two specialisms; nor does it require two years professional experience in nursing prior to the training (DGS/DHOS 2002d).

Specialist and consultant nurses are more recent developments (WHO 2000a:13) that came about from the need in specialised units (for example, neurosurgery, dialysis and oncology) to provide in-service training to new staff at a time of high staff turnover (Dechanoz 1990:158–9). Specialist nursing would have also provided an extended clinical career for these nurses without the need to move into nurse management or the academic field. However, this aspect of nurse specialisation within hospitals appears not to have materialised, for while the training opportunities exist the career structure does not and without official state recognition and regulations there will not be extra pay for this specialist work. However, as the *Infirmier Generale* of a Paris hospital and her colleagues explained (via an interpreter), in March 1998 'Once you are in a specialty you are – you can do much more in a practice – the other thing you can do is - [you] can go further in the hierarchy'. But the movement up the hierarchy would be into nurse management not into a senior specialist post.

Within the UK there has been a considerable interest in the emergence of clinical nurse specialists particularly in infection control, tissue viability, soma care and continence (WHO 2000b: para 3.2.7) – all particular concerns of government for the good reason that there are concerns around the quality of these services. There is also perceived scope for nurse specialists within anaesthetics, outpatient consultations and as surgical assistants (Dowie and Langman 1999). Nurses themselves are a little reticent on the issue, on the grounds that the apparent opportunity presented for greater autonomy and professional status may in practice reflect a poisoned chalice. There are two reasons for this: first, such new and/or extended roles would take them away from their key role of basic care (this resonates with the debate in France and Germany and no doubt other European countries too) and, second, rather than enhancing the changes will mean an extending of their nursing role to take on tasks hospital doctors no longer have the time or inclination to perform (Witz 1995:31).

These issues are rather more complex than they may first appear. First, the arguments for enhancing nursing roles was linked to the Project 2000, the establishment of the UKCC and the concept of new nursing; in short, the move towards nurse education and training went beyond the practicalities of bedside patient care and emphasised much more the intellectual components of nursing. Many within the profession, apparently, were critical of these developments on the grounds that this would divide nursing into an elite graduate profession on the one hand and a larger body of NVQ certificated health care assistants (Walby and Greenwell with others 1994:79). In addition, this change might well mean nursing losing control of the nursing workforce to the human resource management specialists. This was clearly, also, an argument to retain the oral tradition of nursing as a craft, again reflecting a nurse ethos that is deep rooted. Moreover, some doctors have been wary of the new nursing, too, as this quote from a medical consultant cited in Walby and Greenwell (1994:81) illustrates: 'I think nurses can get too much theory...Nurses feel they know best and often there is competition between doctors and nurses, which is unhealthy.' All of which fits into the 'rank-and-file' segment of nursing (see Chapter 2) where the linkage between medicine and nursing is most strongly of the 'handmaiden' variety even if such a terminology is avoided.

The second concern of the nursing profession is that, rather than enhancing the status and autonomy of professional nursing, the nurse specialists will be carrying out routine medical tasks doctors cannot or will no longer carry out. In the UK this was highlighted by the parallel battle of junior hospital doctors for a reduction in their total hours of work per week. This in turn related the settlement between the state and medical profession for part of the implicit understanding between them has been that the number of full-time hospital specialist posts would be kept low relative to other countries (for example, nearly half that of France, see WHO Statistics 2002) but in return the consultants would be treated much the same as the *chef de services* in France (except, unlike their French counterparts, the UK *chef* could also engage in private practice. This elite stratification of the medical profession meant, among other things, that doctors in training (junior doctors) were expected to be on duty for very long hours, probably much longer than anywhere else in Europe. In a deal agreed in 1990 junior doctors' hours on duty would be reduced to no more than 56 hours by 1997 (Dowie and Langman 1999). The real concern of nurses was that all the work not covered as a result would be passed on for the nurses to do. A realistic apprehension, but one that was balanced by the opportunities it presented for nurses wishing to follow a career within clinical nursing. It is a possibility that the introduction of the role of nurse consultants (European Observatory – UK 1999:77) reflects the interests of the state rather than the professionalisation project of nursing, even though it may not be against the nurse professionalisers interests. The point is that it glides over the internal wrangling within the profession. In short, with the shift from medical dominance to managed care it is now in the interest of the state to enhance the career prospects of an elite within nursing. The other example of a state-led initiative has been the introduction of nearly two thousand 'modern matrons' (Department of Health 2000; 2002), which is a role that crosses over the professional leadership and nurse manager role at ward level.

Nurse and hospital management

There has been a nursing directorate headed by the director of nursing (*infirmiéré général*) within all French public hospitals since the Hospital Act, 1991 (WHO 2000a). Very recently, following the decree of 19 April 2002, the role of *infirmiére général* (director of nursing) has been replaced by the *directeur des soins* (director of care). This role now covers allied health professions (réhabilitation), clinical and laboratory services (*medico-techniques*) as well as nursing (*infirmiéres*) and the person carrying out this role may be recruited from any of these occupations (DGS/DHOS 2002e). The expectation must be that the responsibility will usually fall to a senior nurse if only because nurses are the largest single occupational group, responsible for the management of care and the resources on the wards and not quiescent if they collectively believe their interests are threatened. At the ward level, the nursing managers operating in each service are the *cadres supérieurs infirmiers*, who are responsible for patient care.

In UK hospitals the equivalent to the *directeur des soins* is usually the trust nurse executive director (European Observatory – UK 2000, para 3.1.6) with overall responsibility for professional accountability, standards audit and quality of services generally. This provides nursing with a position on the hospital trust board providing professional leadership with a distinctive portfolio cognate with nursing, but without direct responsibility for nursing on the wards. This is configured through the nurse input into the clinical directorates, which are chaired by hospital specialists (that is, consultants) and with an appointed medical director sitting on the hospital board ensuring the medical perspective is taken into account in the decisionmaking processes. In some senses this is not dissimilar to The Netherlands which also focuses on the nurse management input at the ward or service level rather than at the hospital board level, the difference being that the UK NHS have identified a particularly distinctive corporate responsibility that nursing has been able to make its own, quality control.

There has been it would seem a sense that doctors and nurses working at ward and clinical directorate level could work more effectively within the new organisational arrangements of NPM. Rather than working hierarchically the priority has become one of '[g]etting health professionals to work together' (Davies 2000). But to achieve this current NHS thinking has run along the lines that there is also a need for greater professional leadership within nursing at the ward level, hence the introduction of the modern matron, with responsibility for leadership at the operational level of the ward, providing impetus for high standards of care within nursing, In addition, as well as the authority to ensure that administrative and support services for patient care are effective and high quality and, overall, being the beacon within the ward setting that everyone, and especially patients and their families, knows they can turn to for 'assistance, advice and support' (Department of Health 2002:1). If successful the modern matron will be pivotal within hospital organisation, providing authoritative leadership at the front line. So far it is too early to say whether modern matrons will be a success or not and there is a danger that they will become supernumerary unless the nurses themselves (even more than patients) view their role as worth supporting and these matrons are able to work effectively, collaboratively and collegially with their medical colleagues. From a managerial perspective the modern matron makes a lot of sense; the question is whether it is also as attractive professionally. For instance, does it provide the autonomy and status that some nurses will aspire too? Will these matrons be able to ensure sufficiently high intrinsic rewards for nursing work to prevent the high labour turnover in the profession? Will the role be seen as the equivalent (or equal but different) to the hospital consultant? One can guess at some of the answers but whatever they turn out to be it remains likely that the modern matron will become embedded within the NHS hospitals, despite their silly name. It will be interesting to see whether they burgeon as part of the nursing profession or become a side-shoot from it with more in common with a school bursar.

Conclusions: the UK and French state and nursing

It is intriguing that the nursing professions working within two different welfare regimes (corporatist and quasi-liberal) should turn out to share so many similarities. Part of the reason will be that the modern hospital is very similar in organisation across Europe, there is, however, another reason that is specific to the UK and France. Within the configuration of the health care actor-network the state plays a significantly more effective and directive role than in other European countries and in doing so can undercut the dominance of the medical profession in relation to nursing. Moreover, it is seen to be increasingly in interests of both the French and UK Governments to reinforce the hospital nursing organisation because of their central and highly visible role in delivering and co-ordinating hospital care as well as their perceived reliability, as compared to doctors, in following directives, or protocols.

Despite the different histories and welfare regime context there are clear similarities in the trajectory of profession – state relations in relation to medicine and nursing. The general argument present here has been that both states have played an active role in eroding medical dominance within hospitals and generally aimed at reinforcing the concept of the health system as one of managed care. The similarities lie with the ability of these étatist, that is, unitary, states to clearly state their objectives. Their ability to realise them has depended on their particular histories and preceding policies, what Wilsford (1994) has referred to as their 'path dependencies'. Thus, though the government's and/or policy actors within both countries have used the language of NPM, this reflects more a common rhetoric than isomorphism (Pollitt 2001); but this is not just a matter of coincidence, for both countries have had to confront the issue of cost containment within the health sector without loss of regime legitimacy (governmentality) and part of achieving this has entailed reconfiguring the role the medical profession and in the process that of nursing too.

For the nursing profession the changes in jurisdiction and interprofessional boundaries have been viewed with some mistrust. Whereas nurses wish to enhance their curative role and relations with patients, what they feel they have been offered is an extension into the technical territory of medicine. Nevertheless, nurses have taken on these extended roles as a result of the state's intervention. The reconfiguration as between these two health care actors has been mediated substantially by the role of the French and UK states. What is distinctive between the two systems possibly even more than the difference in regime type (neo-liberal hybrid and quasi-corporatist) or, probably, as a consequence of this difference is the relative relationship between general practitioner and hospital specialist. Within France, the general practitioner as a family doctor is a very recent development which has yet to take root in the system. Unlike the British system, patients can access the doctor of their choice. This has led, as with other corporatist systems in Europe, to higher levels of user satisfaction than has been common in the UK. At the same time it has made for a more expensive system. The UK system of general practitioners acting as gatekeepers on the other hand, is in principle a far more rationale system, it should ensure specialist resources are accessed only by patients that require them. However, while the UK looked to adopt NPM solutions within the NHS in the 1980s in order to contain costs, the fact of the matter was that the UK patient was being significantly under-resourced and the government strategy for 'growing' the NHS is to somehow provide a service that is, to quote the rhetoric, 'modern-dependable' but also is reflected in patient satisfaction and voter appreciation. The French state does have to reduce costs of health care and find a way of doing so that does not alienate the patient or the citizen.

5
Germany and Italy: Federalism and Regionalism

Germany and Italy are two countries which are, historically, examples of 'conservative and strongly "corporatist" welfare states' (Esping-Anderson 1990:27) even if this is no longer the case for Italy in the field of health care. Germany is the European country with the strongest *Rechtsstaat* tradition with the state as the point where the federal interests are integrated and underpinned by an extensive legal framework (Pollitt and Bouckaert 2000:53). This contrasts markedly with the Italian political traditions and has implications for the health service in each country as well as their medical and nursing professions. Italy had for over thirty years a nationalised health service, which would seem to suggest it has more in common with the UK model. As will be explained later, this would be an inaccurate assumption for a range of historical, cultural and political reasons. On the other hand, in relation to Germany there is an intriguing symmetry between the two health systems. Germany is formally decentralised (federalism) but subject to *centripetal* forces of increasing federal state regulation. Italy has had a formally centralised health system that is subject to strong *centrifugal* forces of regionalism. On the other hand, the professional organisation of hospital doctors and nurses in the two countries is rather less symmetrical. German hospital doctors accept their professional responsibility and zealously guard their rights of self-regulation. Italian hospital doctors would appear to enjoy less autonomy and are confronted with cross-cutting commitments of a particularistic and clientelistic kind that compromise the profession's ability for self-regulation. The Italian nursing profession appears to have greater autonomy and status than its German counterparts, but the differences between the formal professional organisations and the work situations of nurses within and between the two countries are more complex than they first appear. In order to deal with these and related issues the chapter is organised as follows: (1) health care reforms and organisational changes; (2) professional organisation and work situation of hospital doctors; (3) comparison of approaches to clinical guidelines and related systems of quality control; (4) professional organisation and work situation of hospital nurses; (5) comparison of nursing and medical work within the two countries.

Health care reforms, hospital doctors and organisational change in Germany and Italy

Germany

Hospitals and the health system

Schwartz and Busse (1997:104), writing for an English-speaking audience, explain the logic of the German health system as follows: 'You cannot understand the German health care system if you do not know about federalism and corporatism. Both are fundamental principles of German politics.' To focus on the health system and necessarily oversimplifying the federal structure and corporatist arrangements of the country there are three key aspects to be comprehended. First, each of the states (*Land*) has a constitution that is of necessity consistent with the federal state (*Bundesstaat*) as a whole. This is the Basic Law (*Grundgesetz*). One of the rules embedded within the constitution is that living conditions will be of an equal standard throughout Germany (ibid.). Second, there are the state governments (*Landtag*), whose responsibility includes the provision of extensive hospital facilities within their territory (Knox 1993:136). Third, there are the corporate bodies directly representing the sickness funds, the physicians and dentists. In addition, there is a fourth group, the hospital associations, which perform similar representative functions to the corporate bodies but are not publicly incorporated bodies and therefore have only limited rights in any negotiations.[1] The system of funding and health service delivery functions through a process of regular negotiations between the sickness funds and service providers (Schwartz and Busse 1997).

The three main actors of the health system that the patient has direct contact are the sickness fund, office-based physician and hospital, and each are sharply separated. A particularly distinctive feature of the system is that the office-based specialists provide specialist services which in other systems are provided by hospital outpatient departments for there is a clear is a division between 'stationary' (inpatient) and 'ambulatory' (outpatient) care. Virtually all ambulatory care is provided outside hospitals by specialist doctors who have their own offices and clinics completely separate from hospitals, and patients can visit whichever doctor they choose. This unique division in German specialist health care delivery has had major repercussions on hospital organisation and delivery of care. Hospitals could until recently only provide stationary care and outpatient/policlinic provision was not legally allowed. More recently this has begun to changed, particularly with the introduction of day surgery but also with a growth of pre- and post-inpatient care (European Observatory – Germany 2000:64).[2] The health system is funded for the most part from the statutory health insurance (*GKV – Gesetzliche Krankenversicherung*). This covers nearly 88 per cent of the population including the unemployed and retired. The remaining citizens are privately insured (European Observatory on Health Care Systems – Germany 2000:39–40). The contributions are distributed across 453 sickness funds, which were traditionally divided into two main types: primary funds, which cover most blue- and white-collar employees, and substitute funds (*Ersatzkassen*), open to white-collar workers only. While there are relatively few of these they recruited around two-thirds of white-collar workers (Knox 1993:58). There are also funds for farmers, miners and sailors (Richard and Schönbach 1996:188). The average contribution rate is 13.5 per cent of pre-tax income paid equally by employee and employer (that is, 6.75 per cent each) (European Observatory – Germany 2000:40).

During the 1990s the rules governing the sickness funds were radically changed. The Health Care Structure Act of 1992 (*Gesundheits-Struktur-Gesetz*) introduced the right of free choice of sickness fund including the right to switch between funds from 1996 (similar to The Netherlands reforms – see Chapter 3). The policy makers were hopeful that the reforms would enhance efficiency through competition while at the same time improving membership satisfaction by way of a greater customer orientation (Richard and Schönbach 1996:188). To ensure equality of provision between sickness funds a risk equalisation scheme was also introduced which requires all funds to either contribute to, or receive compensation from, the scheme depending on the demographic (age, sex, employment) composition of their membership.

While the cost-push in health care is similar to other countries (new technologies, changing demography and raised expectations of patients), in Germany the dynamics of cost-containment have been rather different. The Health Care Reform Act of 1989 concentrated on containing the cost of care provided by the independent practitioners (ambulatory care) with the aim of preventing the contribution rates to the sickness funds from rising, for such increases are politically sensitive. Another factor has been the need to comply with Maarstricht criteria, and in 1996 the Federal Minister of Health forced a legal reduction in sickness fund contributions of 0.4 per cent as from January 1997. The Health Care Structure Act, which came into force 1 January 1993, introduced legally fixed budgets for much of the health sector and a partial introduction of a quasi-prospective payment system for the hospital sector (from 1996). Cost-containment measures within health care have focused on organisational reforms designed to rationalise the delivery of services rather than ration them. The aim has been to modernise corporatism not to replace it with new public management (NPM) principles. A significant driver for cost-containment has been the cost of reunification (European Observatory – Germany 2000:51) reflected in the country's health expenditure rising from 8.5 per cent to 10.5 per cent of GDP between 1979 and 1999 (OECD 2000).

Cost containment for the hospital sector (stationary care) through fixed budgets was not a success (Busse and Howorth 1999:321) for, unlike the office (ambulatory) physicians, hospitals stand outside the institutional framework of German corporatism and instead negotiate individually and directly with the sickness funds (Schwartz and Busse 1997:107). The responsibility for hospital planning lies with the local states following the 1972 Hospital Financing Act (KHG).[3] Each state has a hospital plan, which determines the number, type and location of hospital beds. The local states pay the capital costs of all hospitals included in the hospital plans, while the running costs of the hospitals are paid by the sickness funds (European Observatory – Germany 2000:98–9). It is only the public sector hospitals (*Allgemeines Krankenhaus*) that are specifically the responsibility of the states (Altenstetter 1989: 159; 1997:155–7; Schwartz and Busse 1997:107). These constitute over 40 per cent of all hospitals and well over 50 per cent (that is, 57 per cent) of the beds (Perleth and Busse 1998:11). The private 'for-profit' sector is quite a small one providing about 18 per cent of hospitals and only 5.7 per cent of the hospital beds. The main alternative to the public sector is provided by the 'not-for-profit' church sector providing more than 40 per cent of all hospitals and 38 per cent of all beds. The relationship between the public and church sectors is a complex one. On the one hand the hospitals compete to fill beds, for this is how they have earned most of their income. On the other, they both contribute to the hospital plan and patients have the right to attend whatever hospital they choose, paid for by the sickness funds. Hospitals in both these sectors also work together through the State Hospital Association

(*Krankenhausgessellschaft*) to represent their common interests. In addition, the doctors from both sectors work together as members of the Doctors' Chambers (*Ärztekammern*), which provides considerable legal autonomy, status and influence to the profession (Knox 1993:86–7).

As a consequence of the failure of the state to contain hospital costs, some well-informed observers can detect a shift to more federal (*Bund*) control (Schwartz and Busse 1997:114). The lever for this shift was the introduction of a quasi-prospective payment system which is set by the Federal Ministry of Health, leaving only the per diem rates open for negotiation locally. To explain, hospitals had introduced global budgets on a voluntary basis in 1995 as a temporary measure until the new prospective payment system was introduced in 1996. There were two varieties of prospective fees introduced: 'case fees' (*Fallpauschalen*) and 'procedure fees' (*Sonderentgelte*). It is important not to overestimate the extent of these changes for, as was explained by the President of a *Ärztekammer* in a research interview[4] in November 2000, case fees and procedure fees were limited to certain surgical procedures only and the per diem charges still accounted for around 80 per cent of the costs of hospital treatment. This is, however, only part of the story for there have been attempts to change the funding structure of the hospitals even more fundamentally. The traditional structure is that hospitals' running costs will be met by the sickness funds and the capital costs by the states. This is known as the dual system of funding and it has been challenged recently by the central government who wanted to changed the system to a monist one in which all the costs are to be covered by sickness funds (European Observatory – Germany 2000:115). The proposed changes alarmed the medical profession greatly for they threatened to undermine their dominance within the hospital sector and would probably threaten medical jobs too. It was the federal constitution and *Länder*, however, who were the more effective at opposing the change. They were jealous of their suzerain powers over the hospital sector and opposed to any shift to monist funding if it meant that the sickness funds would have the power to determine hospital capacity and not themselves. However, sustained by the German constitution, the *Länder* strongly defended their interests through the *Bundesrat* (the upper house of the German parliament), which has the power to overturn legislation from the *Bundestag* (the lower house). The outcome was that the *Länder* were successful in removing the threat of monist funding even if they have had to accept a more centralised and rigorous cost-containment regime.

The proposed monist system would have been based on a DRG (diagnosis related groups) system planned to be fully operational by 2003. While the principle of dual funding (from state and sickness funds) has been preserved, the policy to introduce DRGs remains. This model has already been tried out within Hamburg public sector hospitals along with other reforms based on quasi-market and NPM principles (Dent *et al.* 2001). This is the largest experiment of its kind in Germany and it is this case study I will focus on here, for it captures a critical moment of change for the country's hospitals and their medical and nursing staffs. It may be that the model will not be adopted to any great extent elsewhere in Germany, although it has already been taken up to some extent by *Vivantes*, the public sector hospital corporation, for Berlin and also in Hanover (Butler 2002), but it does provide a crucial setting for addressing the question as to what are the implications of public management reforms for hospital doctors and nurses in a far more direct way than would be possible elsewhere in Germany.

The Hamburg case

As a consequence of the increasing economical constraints imposed by the health reform in Germany The *Landesbetrieb Krankenhauser* (LBK) (State Enterprise Hospitals for Hamburg) was set up as an autonomous organisation in 1995 with a board (*Vorstand*) of three 'directors'. The hospitals provide just over 6800 beds (LBK 1998) and 'treat...about 108,000 inpatients per year and about the same amount of outpatients per year' according to one senior LBK Manager. The smallest hospital has 235 beds and the largest 1700. The average size is 850 beds; for comparison, the not-for-profit hospitals are all less than 600 and typically between 200 and 250 beds (*Hamburg Krankenhausgessellschaft* 1999). This is consistent with the national figures cited earlier (Perleth and Busse 1998). The group consists of eight acute hospitals supported by about twenty service centres. The LBK 'enterprise' was established principally as a means of reducing costs dramatically through a major rationalisation process. The challenge has been to cut costs by between 25 and 30 per cent between 1996 and 2003. The LBK 'corporation', however, has not been able to use its greater size to negotiate more favourable terms with the sickness funds, only to rationalise the cost structures internally. The official management version of the LBK strategy has been summarised by the chief executive (Lohmann 2000), in a 'Management Letter' (see Box 5.1[5]) which is clearly a managerialist manifesto that challenges the medical dominance traditional within German hospitals.

Box 5.1   Modernity through FIT

Progress   *(Fortschritt)* →**Innovation**   *(Innovation)* →**Teamwork** *(Teamarbeit)*

The programme is in three parts
FIT 1 [P]roductivity. This means about 2,000 reductions in work places...
FIT 2 [T]he slimming down of the range of services...[All] the services that are not patient oriented...are to be taken out of the hospitals...
FIT 3. [H]ospital enterprises that are able to optimise medical processes have the chance to survive...Each hospital will... provide the basic services...Special[ist] services, however, will be restricted to particular hospitals...[T]he aim [is] to standardise the process of treatment...

(Lohmann 2000: 4–7)

Is this the end of medical dominance?

Traditionally at the head of all German hospitals is a triumvirate of directors: nursing, financial and medical director. Formally, as one medical director within the LBK explained, they constitute a *'colleagium*...[of] three people...speaking with one voice'. The medical director, however, is viewed within the profession as 'first among equals'. But the establishment of the LBK as the umbrella organisation, with the responsibility of strategically co-ordinating the management of the eight hospitals, the role of the medical director has changed. The pressures on the collegiate model within these hospitals have increased. As a leading member of the *Ärztekammer* commented, 'The medical director today is the willing instrument [*Erfüllungsgehilfe*] of the executive board internally.[6] No longer is the role one of *primus inter pares* (first among equals) within the LBK. Instead it is emerging as a distinct and separate specialist managerial role. More broadly, the organisational reforms within these LBK hospitals fundamentally question the authority of the medical profession within the hospitals. According to the German federal law, hospitals are organizations under permanent medical direction in order to ensure they fulfil their proper role within the health care system (Hajen, Paetow and Schumacher 1990: para 7.1). Thus medical dominance has been legally embedded within the institutions of

German health care. The managerial changes have considerably reconfigured the role of medical director, translating the notion of the legally
enshrined notion of 'medical direction' from one of professional leadership within the hospital to being the instrument of the executive
board of the LBK. Lest such a change should be viewed as the begin-
nings of a proletarianisation of the German hospital physician it is
worth pointing out that the profession's clinical autonomy remains
strong and is effectively protected, and that the senior hospital doctors
continue to constitute a powerful elite. These are the departmental
chiefs (*Chefärzte*) who are extremely well paid and influential figures
(Knox 1993:103). They also have the right to treat private patients
within the hospitals alongside their other work, although this has been
modified within the LBK so that private patients are paying patients
(*Wahlleistungspatient*) of the hospital and not the doctor. The latter is
rewarded not by private fees but with a performance bonus (LBK 2000).

Within German hospitals generally doctors' career grades have been
usefully described for a British audience as follows:

> The head of department (*Chefarzt*) has ultimate clinical responsibility
> and performs weekly ward rounds on all wards of the department.
> The senior physicians (*Oberärzte*) are specialists who...supervise
> junior staff but do not have ultimate responsibility for clinical care.
> *Assistenzärzte* are the equivalent of specialist registrars. Each ward has
> a ward physician (*Stationsärzt*), who is an *Assistenzärzt* and is respon-
> sible for the day-to-day patient care on that ward. (Maclachlan 1997)

In contrast to the independent office-based practitioners, hospital doctors
are salaried and are represented by the *Marburgerbund*, which functions
as a trade union. It is probably fair to say that discussions of the German
medical profession have tended to emphasise the role of the independent practitioner (office physician) at the expense of the hospital doctors.
The common assumption has been that hospital doctoring is little
more than an apprenticeship for independent practice (Moran and
Wood 1993:69; Knox 1993:85; Moran 1999:115). However, the opportunities for independent practice have significantly lessened over recent
decades and there are now many more hospital doctors than openings
for new office-based practice. Whereas in 1970 there were more independent practitioners (49,827) than hospital doctors (40,172), by 1996
the relationship had more than reversed: 115,538 hospital doctors to
95,271 independent practitioners (Perleth and Busse 1998:12). During
this same period the sickness funds have been given increased powers

(from the 1993 legislation) to refuse new applications if there are, in their terms, sufficient office physicians already in practice. This has meant an increasing number of doctors accepting with some reluctance that their career will be entirely within the hospital sector.

Within the LBK hospitals in Hamburg it is perhaps unsurprising that it is the departmental chiefs (*Chefärzte*) who represent the main source of opposition to the new organisational arrangements. It is not all or even most departmental chiefs, nevertheless the LBK management do from time to time have difficulties in gaining the co-operation of some of them for, while the LBK has the legal right to merge hospitals and departments, individual chiefs can prove to be very uncooperative. In one case, according to one senior manager, it proved necessary '[to] equip...two departments of '[ENT]' surgery in...one hospital, which [wa]s kind of hard to organise...but we made it. Both are in one hospital now'.

This duplication of a specialist service is very much against the FIT principles cited earlier (Box 5.1), but it has concentrated the service in only one hospital. The long-term aim will be to merge the two departments once one of the chiefs retires, but for the moment the strategy is one of attrition and the management are content to wait. This level of resistance, however, is not common, for many doctors have reluctantly come to accept the changes. As a member of the local *Ärztekammer* board (who was also a representative on the LBK board and a *Marburgerbund* activist) explained, 'we...tell our colleague that there's no other way – it's legal[ly prescribed] – it's, it's '*gesetzlich*'...Nevertheless, try to say what is important for your patient and not to save money just for the hospital'. Clearly, the tone is a regretful one and the justification for co-operating with the organisational changes is explicitly and solely based on an acceptance of the legal position.

Clinical Guidelines and Evidence-Based Medicine

Within the German hospital system there has been a relative absence of pressure on hospital doctors to adopt any system of medical audit or clinical guidelines, although this is beginning to change (European Observatory – Germany 2000:91). There does exist the important Committee of Physicians and Sickness Funds, which has issued 16 guidelines over recent decades (ibid:34) but none are *clinical* guidelines; they relate instead to the regulation of prescriptions of pharmaceuticals, medical aids and care by non-physicians. However, there has now been established at the federal level a Committee for Hospital Care introduced under the Reform Act of Statutory Health Insurance 2000 (ibid:35).

This body comprises nine sickness fund, five hospital and four Federal Doctors' Chamber (*Ärztetag*) representatives plus a chairperson from the Federal Committee of Physicians and Sickness Funds, in other words a finely balanced membership between purchasers and providers within which the doctors are numerically in a minority. There is likely to be a further committee established as part of an overall strategy to strengthen the quasi-corporatist status of hospitals and thereby make them more responsive to central direction. Part of its work, it appears, will be to oversee the work of a co-ordinating committee, which will have the responsibility of establishing treatment guidelines and related matters (ibid). This would be the German corporatist equivalent of NICE (National Institute of Clinical Excellence) in the UK and ANAES in France. But whether it will function and do so effectively in relation to the hospital sector is dependent upon whether its quasi-corporatist status is found to be acceptable by the *Länder* and the *Ärztekammern* or not.

Clinical guidelines are not unknown to hospital doctors within the LBK, as the following interview extract with a specialist illustrates.

> Yes, there are clinical guidelines that are introduced by the *Deutsche Gezellschaft* [Scientific Society] for [ENT]...A lot of guidelines...[But] I have no practice with the guidelines. Not at all. I *read* them!...No one asked me to work with the guidelines! (*emphasis in the original*)

A medical director from another LBK hospital explained how it was the practice for the hospital specialists within some hospitals to organise medical audits of their departments where a specialist *Chefärzt* from another city would review a random selection of typically 200 medical records: 'and then this Chief Doctor came for two days, studied these reports, and then he...had the right to interview every...doctor or nurse or whatever he wanted here.' There does not appear to be any legally enforced requirement for this kind of audit, none the less it is a well-established practice if not a necessarily widely practiced one.

Clinical governance in the form of clinical guidelines and evidence-based medicine is a relatively new arrival within the German hospital system and its reception by the medical profession is mediated as much by its members' concerns at the putatively increasing powers of the sickness funds to impose them as it is on their medical judgement as to their clinical value. On balance, however, it is likely that most hospital specialists will find clinical guidelines acceptable so long as they see them as the product of their scientific societies more than the imposition of any federal-level committee for hospital care. To date, however, there is little sign of any organised opposition from the *Ärztekammern* or *Ärztetag*.

Hospital incorporation

The managerial strategy of the LBK has primarily been one that ensures these hospitals fit within the German corporatist framework rather than a radical departure from it, despite first impressions that this was an alien NPM strategy. It is, however, too early to judge this experiment a success (or a failure). Significant, for instance, is the issue of DRGs. The model adopted as the basis for the internal accounting system within the LBK is a US-based system. This is apparently no longer the one that is to be introduced nationally. The newer model, according to a leading member of the *Ärztekammer* is one developed in Australia.

> It...has the advantage that the severity of illnesses are being considered and that different diagnoses are being considered...[O]ne, [of] the disadvantages of...the [previous version of] DRGs, [was] that [it was] much rougher...[and] the relative weight (*Fallgewichte*) and calculation of charges was completely in the stars!

The adoption of a DRG system will perhaps rationalise the financial relations between sickness funds and hospitals, while the new managerialism, to the extent it is taken up across Germany, which may well be quite limited, will undermine the professional dominance of the hospital doctors and especially the *Chefärzte*. But rather than undermining the corporatist institutions these changes will reflect more the reconfiguration of the corporatist system than it being undermined by the any Anglo-American contagion of NPM. The LBK in Hamburg has been a pragmatic pilot for these developments, which are already being implemented in Berlin, and some observers expect them to be 'rolled out' in other *Länder* across Germany (Newbacher and Scheidges 2000). Within the climate of cost-containment, any reorganisation of the hospital sector to better fit the country's corporatist institutional arrangements will mean a tendency towards greater managerial and lesser political control of the hospital sector. The LBK Hamburg provides a critical case that greatly aids our understanding of the dynamics at work within the German hospital sector. Its selection here is precisely because of its difference from, rather than its being representative of, the rest of the country, for the challenges to Hamburg's public sector hospitals epitomises the problems confronted by the public sector hospitals across the country even if Hamburg itself is distinct and different from all or most of the rest of Germany.

Italy

The case of Italy is rather different from Germany in that current reforms are designed to federalise the, previously, formally centralised system of health care. One of the points of interest here is the question as to how far the policy of federalisation will mean the country's health care system and its professions will also become more corporatist? It is impossible to discuss this issue without taking into account the huge differences economically, socially and politically between North and South Italy and the implications these too have had for the health system.

The Italian national health care system was introduced in 1978. The *Servizio Sanitario Nazionale* (SSN) (health care system) was primarily the outcome of Berlinguer's 'historic compromise' (*Compromesso Storico*), a coalition government containing both Christian Democrats and Communists, and reflected a particularly difficult period in Italy's recent history (Fattore 1999:512). The '[L]eft admired the British system for the equality it offered in terms of access as well as finance. The right saw the model as one that offered an effective means for rationing care and reducing costs (Spence 1996:63). Prior to 1978 the health care system and its funding was similar to the German arrangements except that it was by the 1970s plagued by 'serious structural problems' and a 'financial crisis' (European Observatory – Italy 2001:14). The dilemma for the Italian policy makers has been that the centralisation of the health care system (SSN) has not resolved the underlying difficulties that led to earlier crises. The question now is, would the adoption of a federal system overcome the current problems? Before answering it is necessary to describe the SSN system and recent attempts at reform, which were based on the principles of NPM and the quasi-market and would suggest – incorrectly as it happens – a convergence along the British route.

Health expenditure within the Italian public sector (that is, SSN) rose less rather more slowly than that for Germany, from 7 percent to 8.4 percent of GDP between 1980 and 1999 (European Observatory – Italy 2001:50). Health care expenditure as measured by proportion of GDP, however, is high compared to other European countries that have adopted a nationalised system, including the UK and all the other Mediterranean Rim countries.

Organisationally the SSN has been, until recently, strongly centralised. There are three main levels to the organisation: (1) state; (2) regional; (3) local (commune). Following the establishment of the SSN the country was divided into 20 regions, 95 provinces and 8066 communes. The regions were divided into about 659 local health units (*unitarie sanitari locali* – USLs). Here citizens were intended to find under one roof the professionals to provide family and outpatients' clinics and social assistance service (Saraceno and Negri 1994:21). By 1995 the number of local health units had been reduced to 228 with an average catchment area of 250,000 people.[7] At the state level the minister of health has had the responsibility for planning, financing, contracts and the regulatory frameworks for pharmaceutical and medical equipment. Starting in 1997 but accelerating following new legislation in 2000, a process of 'fiscal federalism' has been underway. Now more emphasis is placed on regional taxes to fund health care while the central funding will be used more to even out the resources available and try to ensure all citizens and their families gain adequate – if not equal – levels of care (European Observatory – Italy 2001:35). At the regional level the authorities have the formal responsibility for ensuring the health services in the region were consistent with national policies and priorities to allocate finances down to the local health units equably and to monitor and evaluate their performance. Since 1999 the regional governments have had the responsibility of establishing and managing a process of institutional accreditation for all hospitals (European Observatory – Italy 2001:99). This includes both the regular assessment of the organisational and managerial arrangements and technological systems as well as the quality of medical work.

The reforms that introduced the SSN, however, have never resulted in a system isomorphic with the British NHS. They never managed to remove the 'clientelistic – particularistic' networks that underpinned the Italian welfare state (Saraceno and Negri 1994:21) particularly in the south, which is also characterised by high unemployment and poor economic performance. For instance in 1991, Levy (1996:3) informs us, Northern and Central Italy had a higher per capita GDP than Germany, France or the UK while the Southern regions of the country were very nearly half of that figure. This is coupled with embedded values of familialism and clientelism that these regions share with Greece (and other Mediterranean societies).[8] Putnam (1993) has argued that this is the consequence of the historical lack of 'social capital' reflected in 'norms of reciprocity and networks of civic engagement' (ibid.:181). This evaluation, however, ignores the historical, material and cultural underpinnings to the social embeddedness of the phenomena, which is rooted in a long history of rural poverty and political domination. Ferrera (1996:25) suggests Italy suffers 'a double deficit of "stateness"', first, because the state is unable to adequately control welfare institutions. The regional authorities have been too powerful, as a policy advisor to the *l'olivo* Government (Centre Left and Green coalition) in Rome explained to me in April 2000:

> in Italy the central Government cannot dismiss the region[al health authority]!...The region is constitutionally protected...And [government] couldn't, it [has] *tried* to intervene directly at the level of the local health authority...at which point the regions went...regularly to the constitutional [court]...protesting against interference in their affairs! And...*frequently* the...Court has come out in favour of the regions...So, the power...central Government has...is very limited and that's why...we've moved gradually but inexorably to a situation of saying, 'Well bugger it! Let's give them all the power they want, and then they're going to have to live with it.' (*emphases in the original*)

There would appear to be a degree of inevitability about this devolution of powers given that the central state has long been struggling unsuccessfully with the historical reality of regionalism (OECD 1994:191–2). In the specific case of the health care system it was in early 1992 that certain administrative powers over hospital planning and management were transferred to the regions. This was part of a broader debate on federalism and led to the *Legge Bassanini* (Bassanini's Law), a reform that extended, significantly, powers to the regions (European Observatory – Italy 2001:5–6). The second deficit of stateness Ferrera (1996:24–5) refers to is the inability of the Italian state to protect public institutions from 'partisan pressure and manipulation': [In Italy] the establishment of a national health service has...promoted...a peculiar *collusion* of public and private...the [SSN] staff (even hospital doctors) are allowed great margins of freedom to render services on a private basis, even within the public structures. Moreover, the organisation of the Italian health care system has been plagued with *partitocrazia*, a particularly Italian form of clientelism, which Krause (1996:172) describes as 'rule by [political] parties. All elements of life are politicised, and every person must belong to a political party, and have a sponsor, in order to succeed'. This is no less true of the professions than other sections of Italian civil society, or management, as one director general of a large hospital enterprise (*Azienda Ospedaliera*) in the North of Italy explained in April 2000 (interpreted by an English speaking physician):

> The selection... [of] the public manager... is weak here... and is much... related to the politics and to the parties... Even if we are not completely come back as in the 80s... it still exists. The law says that all the managers... must be chosen from the political board. Of course they must have some professional requirements... [T]here are some good politicians that choose people [with] quality education. Others just choose people that they can trust, [who will] do what they want.

An Italian journalist recently referred to the 'appalling damage that is caused daily by socially accepted corruption in Italian public and private life' (Pacitti 2002:38) even though many have assumed that such practices died with the collapse of the Christian Democrat hegemony in the 1980s. It was the right-wing coalitions of the mid 1990s (*Lega Nord, Forza Italia* [Berlosconi's movement] and the post-fascist National Alliance) that profited electorally from the revelations of widespread bribery (*tangentopoli* – 'bribesville') in politics and the public sector (Fattore 1999:524). But while the more corrupt elements of Italian clientelism may have been dealt with the underlying system of *partitocrazia* would appear to live on relatively unscathed. In Northern Italy it would appear that the practice is probably similar to the 'clientele-relationships between political parties and health sector interest to be found in German local state (*Land*) politics groups' (Giaimo and Manow 1997:185) rather than with the particularistic clientelism associated with Southern Italy. This latter variety can easily take an overtly corrupt form (Ferrera 1996:25), with public goods and services being used for private ends, although it is not necessarily corrupt but a means of coping with uncertainty through a network of loyalties and obligations. In Southern Italy it is the continuing relevance of a strong Catholic Church and family-centred local society – a Catholic subidiarity (Ferrera 1996:30) that provides the underlying legitimation while the considerably higher levels of poverty and unemployment ensure its continuation (ibid: 21–2; Piattoni 1998).

Once in office the right wing coalition of Berlusconi adopted a Thatcherite approach to the implementation of the health care reforms introduced by the previous administration. Parliament finally approved the 'framework' Bill in 1992 (amended in 1993). It was cost containment (even more than ideology) that then dominated the health policy agenda (Fattore 1999:522–4). The reforms were driven in large part by the pressure of the Maarstricht Treaty to reduce public expenditure (Ferrera 1995:299; Fattore 1999:523–4). In this respect they were expected to take the politics out of health care delivery. The 1992 reforms consisted of three main themes (ibid:532):[9]

1 *Decentralisation.* The national government remained responsible for overall funding and defining the services provided by the SSN but the regions now had the responsibility of ensuring that a minimum range of services was provided. They also had the task of rationalising the delivery of health care at the local level. As a consequence the original 659 local health units reduced and reorganised to become 228 health authorities (*Aziende Sanitarie Locali*). A number of hospitals also achieved self-governing status including all the university hospitals, which meant they too came under regional control.
2 *The quasi-market.* The two terms 'competition' and 'market' were never used by the legislators when drawing up 1992 reforms. Nevertheless, the new funding rules for hospital and specialist care suggested a potential for competition for patients and resources between public and private providers (Ferrera 1995:276).[10] Within the public sector overt marketisation has had much less influence than managerialism with its emphasis on efficiency and effectiveness.
3 *Managerialism.* The reforms replaced consensus management with managerialism. Within the hospitals this meant the introduction of the director general. The intention was that this new species of manager would be chosen according to their managerial experience and education rather than patronage. Two senior managers would support and advise the director general, the medical and administrative directors (note the absence of a nursing director, a point to be returned to later). All these changes were intended to provide clear lines of accountability within the hospital and with the health authorities. The 1992 reform also introduced the Council of Health Professionals, a consultative body for the director general (Fattore 1999:534). This body represented all health professionals but medical doctors made up the majority of elected representatives.

It was managerialism rather than marketisation that had the most significant impact. The goal overall was to contain costs further reinforced by the 1999 reforms (European observatory 1999:16). This new managerialism, is a decentralised one reflecting the traditional regionalism of the country, but the centre is not without influence and was, for example, able to introduce DRGs in 1995[11] along with the requirement that regions fund public and private hospitals according to a prospective per-case payment system (Fattore 1999: 536). Regions have the power to set up their own system but they cannot exceed fees laid down by the national scheme. Nevertheless, despite the 'success' of DRG implementation the double deficit of stateness (Ferrera 1996: 25) continues to undermine the possibility of a uniform national health service and raises the question whether the reforms are able to move the system towards a German 'federal' model. The problem here, however, is that Italy lacks the institutional and legal framework that buttresses the decentralism of federalism with a strong enough national identity to ensure policies of social solidarity and inclusion are also effective. In Germany the challenge was the incorporation of the East German *Länder*, in Italy it is the 'Southern Question' (*La Questione Meridionale*) and of the two it is the latter that has proved to be the more intractable. Moreover, rather than resolving the question, current policies would seem to be exacerbating them.

The organisation of the medical profession

The *ordini* are the state regulatory bodies through which the professions are expected to regulate themselves and to advise government. They are formally intended to function in a way parallel to the *Ärtzekammern* and there is a national *ordine* federation for doctors in Rome. *Ordini* were first formed in 1874, initially for lawyers, the *ordine* for the medical profession was established in 1910 (Krause 1996:174).[12] They are semi-public (that is, corporatist) regional organisations run by the profession with which all qualified doctors must register in order to practice. Italian doctors, however, are equivocal about their *ordine* because it is seen as a state imposition and has greater relevance to the functioning of *particrazia* than to their professional work.

It is the 'scientific societies' that would appear to be providing an alternative network within the profession, especially among those working within university hospitals, and they could emerge as an important source of expert advice on clinical guidelines and related developments (following the 1999 reforms). Unlike their German counterparts, however, the professional identity of the Italian hospital doctors is an equivocal one, particularly within the public sector where their careers structure is much more managerial than has been the case in most of the rest of Europe. This and the cross-cutting commitments of a particularistic – clientelistic kind have compromised the profession's ability for self-regulation.

The way that many hospital doctors sought autonomy and status was through private practice for, as one hospital specialist from Southern Italy commented to me in March 2000, 'In the past we didn't care because we got money from the private patient.' All or much of this is now changing.

Hospital doctors' work situation

Hospital doctors are still able to opt for part-time contracts (as in Britain) and reclaim autonomy by engaging in private practice. Within Italy, however, private medical practice is a most competitive activity, for there are 5.5 doctors per 1000 population (WHO Statistics 2002), which is the highest figure in Europe. This figure reflects, in important part, the dominant influence and interests of the universities within government with the result that there has been a virtual absence of any effective limit to the numbers of medical students (*numerus clausus*) (Krause 1996:178).[13] The comparable figure for Germany is 3.5 per 1000 population, which is more or less a median figure for the Continent. This overproduction of medical doctors has had real implications for the organisation and management of nursing work (see below).

Hospital physicians are salaried and divided into first-level and second-level physicians (*dirigente medico di primo livello* and *dirigente medico di seconda livello*). The senior physician in charge of the hospital unit defines the duties of the first-level doctors. The more senior, second-level doctors will be responsible for the medical management of patients as well as having management duties in relation to the hospital unit (European Observatory – Italy 2001:89). Between 1992 and 1999 hospital doctors could also have their own 'fee-for-service' private practice outside the hospital. The organisational arrangements between 1978 and 1992 seriously constrained doctors' autonomy, with medical work being organised strictly along civil service rules with seniority being the key to promotion (Freddi 1989:20). The 1999 reforms associated with the National Health Plan for 1998–2000 (European Observatory – Italy 2001:96) would appear to be moving the pendulum back in that direction, although not quite. Hospital doctors can still choose to treat private patients but only, in principle, within the public hospital, where between 6 and 12 per cent of beds should be reserved for the purpose (European Observatory – Italy 2001:100). Some private practice outside the hospital is still permitted for doctors appointed before 1998 but they can only, formally, be on a part-time contract with the SSN and, moreover, they have to accept that their hospital careers will be limited by this choice (European Observatory – Italy 2001:100).

In practice this is not always the case, as one senior physician from Southern Italy explained, in March 2000, in answer to the question 'do you see your private patients in the hospital?': 'No, I receive [them] in my private office, but with the permission...[and] on behalf of the hospital.' This was not an exceptional case and it would appear that hospital managements were considering allowing this practice on the grounds that the hospitals did not provide the environment private patients expected. It is unlikely, however, that this reflects the kind of 'attrition' strategy noted in the case of the German managers rationalising clinical services in Hamburg. It would seem unlikely for the present that the practice will die out although one can anticipate that there will be considerable variation across the country reflecting the new federalisation as well as the traditional regionalism of the country. It would appear that the hospital managers are attempting to respond to public (and doctors') demand for private practice while at the same time extending greater control over medical work. Unlike the German situation there is no strong sense of corporate ideals of 'responsible autonomy', *partitocrazia* still appears to exercise a corrosive influence that prevents a more virtuous form of subsidiarity emerging.

Clinical guidelines

The other issue concerning the work situation of doctors to be addressed here is that of quality assurance and clinical governance. The National Health Plan for 1998–2000 introduced a national programme on health care quality whose objectives included, importantly, a system of institutional accreditation for public and private providers and the establishment a national programme on clinical guidelines (European Observatory – Italy 2001:102). These policies extended other quality initiatives of the early 1990s aimed at improving users experience of the health care system in a similar way to the Patients Charter in the UK (European Observatory – United Kingdom 1999:36–7). The issue of clinical guidelines, however, is particularly interesting because it has become the ubiquitous instrument of clinical governance that impinges on the day-to-day work of hospital doctors. This is not to pretend that clinical work is now wholly dictated by guidelines – it is not – but increasingly elements of the work processes are being codified with the expectation that practitioners will learn, internalise and practice them.

The concerns for the Italian hospital doctors, as much as for any others, have been (1) are they driven by the need to improve care or the efficient use of resources?; and (2) Do they maintain the clinical autonomy of the hospital specialist? For example, in one hospital in

Central Italy the medical director reported that their policy was to concentrate attention on developing clinical guidelines based on the five most commonly used DRGs. This would have the effect of both improving the consistency of care and the efficient use of resources. It would also challenge the conventional wisdom of clinical research, which is to study the 'interesting cases' that are by definition uncommon in favour of the routine. Nevertheless, the legal imposition of clinical guidelines has not generally been met with hostility from within the profession. For the 'scientific societies' (as mentioned earlier) the development may mean an enhanced role for them. For the individual hospital specialist the prospects are mixed; for example, a typical response provided by a specialist in internal medicine from southern Italy in March 2000: 'generally we...practice medicine without using our guidelines. We remember what we have learnt at the university, or what we learn by means of scientific publications but we are not particularly...interested in [the] uniform...practice of medicine.' But a colleague of this same physician, on a separate occasion, commented that while 'in some cases it is true that we are restricted by the use of guidelines but, on the other hand, many colleagues are protected by using these guidelines'. These two physicians, it has to be added, were responsible for overseeing the introduction of clinical guidelines and audit within the hospital. They nevertheless are a fair representation of the attitudes of the hospital specialists, for as a specialist gynaecologist also remarked '[in] my opinion...physicians now underst[an]d that in litigation to have guidelines...is a shield.

Although it is important to recognise there are others who are less convinced of the merits of clinical guidelines, such as this professor of medicine from Northern Italy, interviewed in March 2000:

> I don't like [clinical guidelines]...for me each patient is a kind of...little war, you cannot generalise...[if] they are very old they accumulate several pathologies, heart disease, lung disease, diabetes, hypertension, and...the guidelines are for a typical or hypothetical patient, not for a patient like this.

In other words, clinical guidelines could be routinising medical work, a viewed not shared by a colleague who emphasised more the importance of their evidence base: 'It's very important to have guidelines, internal guidelines based on what is recognised by the scientific community.'

Generally, across Italy, hospital specialists are working on developing and implementing clinical guidelines often with the mixed objectives of improving care and economic efficiency. There is some debate around whether the scientific associations should play a more central role in this process, although for the most part the guidelines are constructed locally from Internet searches of North American and possibly British literature (the approach varies between hospitals). The general impression one is left with is that many Italian doctors are experiencing the implementation of clinical guidelines as some kind of compensatory mechanism for weak professional organisations. After all, it is they who have to organise and implement them and while they are closely constrained my managerial concerns for efficiency this is nothing new. Rather than encroaching on clinical autonomy there is a perverse sense in which clinical guidelines may be expanding it.

German and Italian hospital doctors: résumé

The Italian health system has been undergoing a process of federalisation over recent years. While these 'centrifugal forces' have been beginning to change the system to one with some parallels to the German model the position of the hospital doctors has not significantly changed. The Italian hospital physician is the nearest version of the proletarianised medical professional in Europe. The hospital organisation within the SSN has always been highly bureaucratised along civil service lines (Freddi 1989:20), careers within the health service are compromised if they also carry out private practice and their professional organisation (*Ordine*) has little authority. Physicians enjoy status as individuals, as university professors advising government or as successful private practitioners. In comparison, the German hospital doctors have a strong sense of professional autonomy reflected in the role and authority of their professional organisation, *Ärztekammern*, and nationally, the *Ärztetag*. Within the hospitals the work situation of the doctors has been hierarchically collegiate with the medical chiefs (*Chefärzt*) wielding considerable influence. This may well be beginning to change with the medical director coming through as the more dominant figure reflecting a growing managerialism within public sector hospitals. This should not be overstated at this stage for the case discussed here (Hamburg) is an early innovator and other states may not follow suit.

In the case of Germany, it is the centripetal forces of centralisation, intended to defend the corporatist traditions against the encroachments of neo-liberalism, that is experienced as undermining local autonomy associated with federalism. For the doctors, the imposition of DRGs and the perceived greater power of the sickness funds have led them to feel a loss of autonomy and status. In addition, the closing off of the opportunity to move into private/independent practice for the majority of hospital physicians has markedly exacerbated this sense of loss. Perversely, however, some doctors view clinical guidelines as a means of improving their professional status. In place of traditional individual clinical practice is the more collectivist organisation of guidelines, which is also seen as creating a potential for a greater role for the scientific societies. The issue of private practice in Italy is more complex, because the rules are being interpreted flexibly in parts of the country so that doctors can continue to see patients privately – in their own offices outside the hospital – so long as these patients are formally accounted for as if they had been seen as paying patients within the hospital. This possibility is not open to German hospital doctors (although it is the case that the medical chiefs can and do see private patients within the hospital).

What is missing from this account so far is the other half of the division of hospital labour, the work and professional organisation of the nurses and their role in the configuration of German and Italian hospital care.

Nurse work and professional organisation

The general lack of professional status for nursing in these two countries has been a consequence of a number of factors, not least the gendered role of women as 'wives and mothers' (Trifiletti 1999:54) rather than 'workers'. This is further reinforced by the culturally embedded notion that nursing reflects a female dedication to a religious ideal. Both of these relate to the values of subsidiarity and familialism which undermines attempts at professionalisation in the cases of female dominated occupations. But there is another more prosaic reason for the failure to professionalise and this is the overproduction of doctors. However, despite the obstacles, there is evidence that the organisation and status of nursing in these two countries is changing and in the process questioning assumptions of what we mean by professionalisation.

Professional organisation

Germany

It was Pastor Fliedner and his wife who created the German nurse. In 1836, the pastor conferred on them the ecclesiastical status of 'deaconess' on them and the organisational principle of the 'Mother

House' (Quinn and Russell 1993:89). It was Agness Karll who, in 1903, who founded the first national 'professional' nurses organisation. There are approximately 750,000 nurses and midwives (WHO 2000d:8), 82 per cent female, with around 50 per cent being employed in the acute hospitals, mainly in the public sector. As in most other European countries there is a shortage of nurses and in the early 1990s, in an attempt to improve recruitment and equalise pay scales across the reunified country, nursing salaries were increased by between 10 and 30 per cent in the Western part of the country and 80 per cent in the East.

General nurse training, as in Italy and elsewhere within the EU, takes three years, and entrance requirements are relatively low, involving completion of school education only. Nursing specialisation (post basic education) is a further two years on in-service training. There are also short courses on ward management and two-year programmes for nursing management and education. There already exist a number of degree courses in nursing management, nursing education and nursing science. These are comparable to a Master's degree (ibid.:12), and since 1998 nursing doctorate programmes have been available. Unlike medicine, the status of nursing as a profession is more linked to its members' claims to academic certification than clinical reputation.

German nursing appears to have a strong professional basis in its educational programmes and this is further reinforced by its professional organisation, the German Nursing Association[14] (*Deutscher Berufsverband für Pflegeberufe-DBfK*). However, this body has no legal role as a professional body as nurses are not officially viewed as a profession and are therefore not organised into 'chambers' (*Kammern*) at the *Land* level (European Observatory – Germany 2000:27) and for this reason do not themselves maintain a register of nurses, this being the responsibility of the public authorities (*Länder*) (Quinn and Russell 1993:91), and membership of the *DBfK* is optional. However, the organised profession of nursing does appear to be having some success in gaining a legally recognised system of representation at the national level. This includes the creation, in 1998, of the German Council of Nursing, a body that 'co-ordinate[s] the political work of several nursing associations and specialist groups' (WHO 2000d:10) and has as its principle aim the establishment of a legally recognised self-governing body for nurses (ibid.:15).

Italy

Italian nurses have also not enjoyed full professional status, although this is in the process of changing. In other words, for the moment they do not yet have their own *ordine*; instead they are organised as a federation of 98 colleges (*collegi*). These were established in 1954 and co-exist with Catholic associations that have an even longer history.[15] There are about 320,000 nurses in total with more than half employed in the private sector.[16] Italian nursing has attracted a higher proportion of men than in most other parts of Europe. Salvage and Heijnen (1997:74, Figure 5) indicate that about 25 per cent of the nursing workforce is male. This is substantially higher than any of the other countries included in this study. Moreover, the distribution of male nurses is particularly concentrated in Southern Italy (Pratschke 2000:6, fn. 5) where a career in nursing offers security of employment, status and even levels of pay that are attractive relative to the other possibilities within the labour market.

The state depends on the *collegi* to maintain the professional register and enforce the code of practice (ethics). The change that is currently underway is one that will upgrade nursing from *collegi* to *ordine* status, which also reflects the extension of nurse education to degree level (*laurea*). This is the outcome of the implementation of the European Community directives on the subject of nurse education and training. Since 1996 the universities have delivered nursing courses.[17] originally the intention had been to close all the nursing colleges and relocate the diploma courses as well as the nursing degree courses (*laurea*) within the universities alongside the medical schools. The nurses' *collegi* fought this move on the grounds that it would deter people coming forward to train because it would mean travelling further away from home and the universities could only provide a limited number of places. In Rome, for instance, the nurses' 20 nursing colleges were retained.[18] The basic nurse training and entry requirement remains a three-years diploma (this too is in the process of change in order to meet EC requirements). It is envisaged that in future it will be possible to undertake an extra two years study to convert the diploma into a degree and this will be the route to take only for those wishing to become nurse directors or teachers.[19] The struggle of nurses for professional recognition will not, however, be resolved with the establishment of a nursing *ordine* coupled with the nursing degree. What is more likely to happen is that nurse managers, teachers and researchers (academics) will become a professionalised segment, or segments, within nursing.

Work situation

There are 2.96 nurses per 1000 population in Italy (WHO Statistics 2002) with only Greece returning a a lower figure. The figure for

Germany is 9.6, which is the third highest in Europe. For those nurses working within the acute hospital sector, the patterns of working and the strategies for attaining greater work autonomy have been rather different within Italian and German hospitals. In general terms, Italian hospital nursing remains doctor-led, predominantly task based and, particularly in the South, rooted in an oral tradition – although this is in a process of change. In Germany, by contrast, nursing work within hospitals has been developed much more self-consciously as a professional, knowledge-based, autonomous activity separate from medicine, and often in conflict with doctors. The differences between the two countries should not be overstated. Substantial as they are, they do appear to be moving along similar pathways towards – possibly idealised – common goals of legally recognised professional autonomy within a clearly demarcated jurisdiction (Abbott 1988). For historical and political reasons Italian nurses have pursued a strategy of seeking state recognition while German nurses have focused more on the workplace situation. Why this is the case is explained in the following sections.

Germany

Nursing work within German hospitals has developed far more as an autonomous activity, separate from medicine and focused on patient-centred care than in the case of Italy. Nursing records for individual patients, for instance, are well established, as is the organisation of nursing according to the principle of 'primary nursing'. A nursing director from a Hamburg public sector hospital in May 2000 described the process of its introduction in the following terms:

> When I started [here about six years ago] most of the wards were doing...functional method [task-based nursing]...I had...to change this kind of method into a more patient oriented method and one of the systems – we call it the 'Room Nursing'...it is Primary Nursing.

What is being described here is the adoption and adaptation of the principles of the nursing process (for example, Paul and Reeves 1995), which parallels the medical processing of the patient. It is a self-consciously professionalising approach that has developed within the English-speaking world, especially but not solely in North America. There are many variations to the basic model but in essence it consists of the following. There is a separate nursing assessment and diagnosis providing the basis for a care plan. This is then implemented and finally evaluated (ibid.:17). The nurse who takes responsibility of carrying out – or overseeing – this process is the 'primary' nurse.

The emergence of primary nursing highlights some important aspects of nursing jurisdiction. The struggle to win independence from doctor-driven work (medical dominance) on the wards did lead to a degree of acrimony between the professions. This is discernible in the following extract from a letter sent by two medical lecturers from Munich and published in the *British Medical Journal* in 1995:

> Whereas a considerable proportion of German nurses, especially in larger hospitals, previously incorporated taking blood, inserting catheters, and giving antibiotics and blood products into their daily duties, they are now unwilling to take on these additional roles. Organising patients' appointments and investigations [are] not considered to be their responsibility. In addition, nurses are now reluctant to dress wounds and remove stitches, even on surgical wards. These jobs have to be delegated to final year [medical] students, who spend their time doing whatever the nurses believe is not their job. (Nikol and Huehns 1995:873)

In order to clearly distinguish nursing from medical work a settlement was arrived at in which nurses concentrated on the organisation and delivery of care completely separately from all technical aspects of medical treatment. This was an arrangement that would seem to limit the possibilities for nurse specialist roles in intensive care, and similar technologically based work, and is a development that contrasts with the situation in North America and Britain where such enhanced roles have, in part, emerged as a means of substituting medical staff input. The position in Germany, however, is not as clear cut as the letter in the *BMJ* suggests, as a senior nurse from a surgical ward explained in May 2000:[20]

> [Nurses] do a lot of things that are supposedly done by doctors, like drawing blood and changing the bottles for chemotherapy and this kind of thing...which actually is doctors stuff. So they do a lot of things because the doctors don't have the time and they take it for granted that nurses are doing it now and that seems to be a source of problems.

Clearly, the struggle to extend and enhance nurses' roles within the hospitals has been a difficult one. Interestingly, one outcome appears to have been a burgeoning of nurse led quality assurance work, is contrast to Italy, where the work is typically done by a doctor (who otherwise might be underemployed).

Italy

Until relatively recently nursing work in Italy has been constitutionally task based. Until six years ago nurses' duties were legally prescribed by the state and listed in a document known as the *Mansionerio*.[21] While this guaranteed them jurisdiction of a sort, it gave them little autonomy. The nursing profession long desired and demonstrated to get that particular law overturned. According to one *collegi* activist (with the aid of an interpreter) from Rome in March 2000, 'We had a big demonstration the first of July...1994...the fight to be...responsible as a nurse.' The *Mansionerio*, however, was not finally abandoned until 1999 and the change has given individual nurses the possibility to develop professional practice and in the process ensured the *collegi*, as the nurses' 'professional' body, have become more influential. This reform, however, has not translated into changes in working practices to any great extent. There are two main reasons for this, both mentioned earlier, the shortage of nurses and the oversupply of doctors, as one senior neurology nurse from Rome, in March 2000, expressed the problem: 'we have a problem...doctors, doctors...loads of doctors and few nurses...There is one nurse for one doctor...in my hospital. Yes, sometimes two doctors for one nurse.' This has meant that much nursing work is in practice carried out by doctors. Even with the surfeit of doctors, however, there are still too few nurses across most of Italy, with Southern Italy as the exception to this rule according to a deputy director of nursing in southern Italy in March 2000: 'we have a lot [of nurses] because until...three years ago you didn't need a diploma to [become] a nurse...So every family who doesn't have money [to send their children to university or college]...they make nurse'. In other words, nursing is viewed as a good alternative to unemployment or working within the grey or black economy, for as this person explained, '[while] in the north [of Italy] you can work in the industry, you can choose. Here you don't have any choice if you don't...study, if you don't have money [you can become a nurse]...It is...only three years – so it is not so difficult...It is not well paid but it is a good job'. This may well explain why it is here, in the South, unlike elsewhere, that the many of nurses are male (Pratschke 2000:6 fn. 5). This also relates to the second issue, the nurses' backgrounds and expectations. Most rank-and-file nurses are content (or at least consent) to carry out task-based, doctor-devolved work and display little interest in extending their role professionally. This can be usefully illustrated with reference to a national project to introduce written nursing records for each individual patient based on a nursing assessment. This three-year project, which started in 1999, is a major challenge, particularly in the South, because, as the assistant director of nursing explained:

> Our nurse[s], they are...thinking only with [the] 'hand'...They are not yet [taking] responsib[ility for] the work...[It is] most difficult for her...to make the change in the mind [to realise]...'OK, you are nurse but you can work in a different way'...Now you have the total order [responsibility] of the 'sufferant' [patient]

Elsewhere in Italy adaptation to the new method of working appears to have been easier to achieve, as a cardiology nurse from a hospital in Central Italy explained: '[We] are...mak[ing] a schedule for each patient...where everybody [that is, nurses] writes what they have done for the patient...and this...goes in the *cartella* [patient record folder].' This – new – nursing record is part of a professionalisation project as much as it is designed to improve patient care (although the two might be assumed to be synonymous), but to be successful it has to be a legal requirement as would be the case in any country with a *rechtstaat* tradition. For the moment nursing records are not a legal requirement, as another nurse (intensive care) from the same hospital explained: 'The law is not very clear...the nurse [notes]...[do] not yet [have] a legal recognisance...[and it is the *collegi's*] objective is that...[it] will...and also the hospital directory [senior management] would wish that [too].' Possibly, once the three years project has been completed, 'legal recognisance' will follow. For the present purpose the point of interest is the difference in approach between the hospital nurses in Southern and Central Italy.

Until recently there were no directors of nursing with a place on the board of management of hospitals and without them the leadership for nurses was missing. Even now it is rare, as the following quote from an interview with the president of one of the *collegi* in March 2000 makes clear: '[The *collegi*] is fighting so that nurs[ing] can have a higher position in the directory [that is, senior management] of a hospital. Until two, three months ago it was impossible for a nurse to be a director at a second level in a hospital...There is [now] the first...Italian nurse [director], who has a contract.' Second level means equal status with the medical director and administrative director. The first level is the director general. Only with a presence within senior management will nursing have the necessary influence to implement nursing reforms within the hospitals.

German and Italian nursing – compared

In some ways the Italian and German nursing professional projects are a mirror image of each other. Italian nurses are well on the way to achieving full professional legal status as an *ordini* on a par, formally at least, with doctors, architects and engineers. German nurses are not legally recognised as a profession. On the other hand, education and training is of a high standard already, achieving what Italian professionals are only now aspiring too. It is within the work situation (reinforced by good levels of education and training) that German nurses have been able to provide themselves with a professional identity and the greatest opportunity for professional development. In Italy, by contrast, hospital nursing is often task based and doctor led and, compared to Germany, is a 'late developer'. These differences reflect the peculiarity of the institutional context that shapes the strategies of the organised nursing profession in the two countries. In part this relates to differences in the configuration of the medical jurisdiction in the two countries and the implications this has for nursing (Abbott 1988:71–2). In Italy the overproduction of doctors has meant that there has been no internal impetus to extend or enhance nursing work. German nursing has, in a sense, been more fortunate in that medical jurisdiction is clearly and legally defined, leaving a clear space for nursing care to develop independently from medicine. For the Italian nurses, by contrast, the elevation nursing from *collegi* to *ordini* is an opportunity the organised profession would be unable to resist. Perhaps with the additional political weight they will be able to ensure reforms in education and training, and nursing process will be consolidated within the hospitals. This may become more likely when the nursing director joins the medical director on the hospital directorate – as in Germany.

The implications for nursing management in these two countries are fairly clear. Until nursing work has independence from direct medical dominance it is difficult to develop effective nurse management systems. It is, however, not only subordination to medicine that leads to inertia within nursing, for the labour market and cultural expectations also shape what is organisationally possible. In Italy, especially in the South, innovations in nursing have had a slow and fitful start, whereas in Germany this is not the case and with the relatively recent settlement between medicine and nursing German nurses are now able to organise and manage their own work within a clearly set out legal framework.

Germany and Italy: comparisons and conclusions

As set out in the introduction the organisation of the health systems in these two countries would appear to be moving in opposite – and possibly converging – directions, a consequence of centripetal and centrifugal political forces; one, Germany, possibly moving more towards state regulation, the other, Italy, certainly moving along a route of greater decentralisation and regionalism towards federalism. An initial question is whether this reflects the global impact of new public management or not? The answer to be derived from the evidence is that it is not, or not entirely so. In Germany what appears to be an NPM style of management reforms are beginning to be adopted with public sector hospitals (*Allgemeines Krankenhausen*), at least in Hamburg and Berlin. However, and intriguingly, instead of evidencing an erosion of corporatism it is precisely the opposite: a corporatist adaptation to changing conditions and underlying pressures. Thus the move to managerialism within public sector hospitals is a strategy of first incorporating them within the corporatist and legal framework, as has always been the case with the office physicians (ambulatory care), and by that process more effectively exercising a policy of cost containment properly. However, in achieving this the *Länder* have to accept a certain loss of autonomy over this sector although it is clear from the discussion on dualist and monist funding that these state governments are very reluctant to give up their role within this sector.

In the case of Italy, the constitutional weakness of the central state has always created problems and particularly so for the health system. Unlike the unitary and bureaucratic model of the UK national health system, the Italian version was constantly being pulled apart by regional opposition to central government policies and frequently challenged through the constitutional courts. In addition, there was the insidious erosion of legitimacy by the effects of *partitocrazia* and, more particularly in the South, clientelism. If the country were to adopt a more federal rather than fragmented structure, and if the health system reflected more a legally framed corporatism as in Germany, it might be possible that the more inefficient and corrupting elements within the system might be driven out. The effectiveness of such a strategy assumes that the Southern European model is more a variant of conservative corporatism (a point to be pursued further in the chapter dealing with Greece and

Poland), whereas it may well be a distinct variety of its own – in which case the move to federalism will result not in a political and social corporatist consensus but possibly the hardening of socio-economic and political divisions between North and South.

As to the issues relating to the medical and nursing professions and their responses to hospital and related reforms, there is again symmetry of opposites. The difference between the professional organisations of doctors in the two countries reflects the different roles of the state in each. In Italy the central government tried to establish control early on in the country's modern existence while in Germany the local state governments enjoyed ascendancy. Formally, the doctors' chamber and *ordine* ensure that all practicing doctors are registered and regulated. In practice, the German doctors are more likely to view the doctors' chamber as a focal point for their professional identity and as their representative organization for lobbying within the political networks. This is not the case with the medical *ordini* in Italy, which shares more in common with the *l'Ordre des Médecins* in France and the Pan Hellenic Medical Society (*Panellionios Iatrikos Sillogos*) in Greece in being experienced by physicians generally as an imposition rather than a body for professional representation. There is some indication that the scientific societies will perhaps take on a greater role in advising the public authorities on medical matters, which may counterpoint the role of the medical *ordini*, for example around the issue of clinical guidelines. Intriguingly, it appears that Italian hospital doctors, despite certain reservations, view the introduction of these guidelines in a positive light. It legitimates rather than undermines their clinical autonomy and possibly offers protection against criticism and litigation. For the German hospital physician, whose clinical autonomy is far more strongly embedded, may well have stronger reservations over their introduction.

In the case of hospital nursing it is interesting but deceptive to note that the German profession remains outside the corporatist framework of the *kammern* (chambers) while the Italian nurses are embracing the opportunity for promotion from *collegi* to *ordini* even if it is doubtful that the physicians, managers or even the general public will view the change in the same way. It is, formally at least, part of the country's response to the demands of the EC for common standards across Europe and in the process the raising of the standards of education and training. Nevertheless, it is in notable contrast to the situation within Germany, where nursing would seem to be restricted in its claim to professional status. While the formal status is a lowly one, the education and training and working conditions of nurses in Germany do appear to be markedly better than in Italy. What is noticeable, however, is the profession's rejection of any extended role that takes them, as they see it, into the territory of the medical profession. To pursue this issue of 'territory' or jurisdiction (Abbott 1988) further it is possible to summarise the comparisons between the two countries in terms of relative jurisdictional power of the medical profession and its practitioners vis á vis management and nursing. In the case of Italy the doctors' jurisdiction has been weak, not because of the power of the state (as in France) but that of the universities. The consequent overproduction of medical graduates has, in turn, limited the prospects of nurse professionalisation by denying the latter the opportunity for any expanded role within the hospital. In contrast, the German physicians have enjoyed a legally and constitutionally underpinned professional jurisdiction. This has limited, or delayed, the encroachment of managerialism within the hospital sector and reinforced the assumption that nursing is primarily an adjunct to medical work rather than a partner in the delivery of health care. Much of this is now changing and, in the case of hospital doctors, precipitated by their inability to move on into independent office practice (ambulatory care) because, similar to Italy, there has been an overproduction of medical graduates. Clearly, medical un- and underemployment erodes jurisdictional power and it seems that the relationship with nurses now is a consequence of some considerable resistance by the latter to medical assumptions of their working relations. But for the nurses, their professional jurisdiction is not constitutionally underpinned at the level of the *Land* and they do not have their own *kammern*. Instead, their jurisdiction is being reinforced by their growing presence within the senior management of hospitals, a strategy the Italian profession is also pursuing, as well as gaining an organised 'voice' nationally.

6
Poland and Greece: Transition or Embeddedness?

In this chapter I describe and compare the Polish and Greek health systems and their medical and nursing professions, and the implications of their position on the periphery of Europe. The notion of periphery being used here not only refers to geography but has another meaning too: Poland was part of the post-1945 Soviet Empire and Greece has strong links with the Balkans and strong Orthodox religious traditions (Mouzelis 1986); both lie outside the welfare regimes identified by Esping-Andersen (1990) and yet are, or are about to be, part of the European Union. Economically neither country is yet in the same league as the other countries discussed in this book. This is, in part, but not solely, because they have been politically and industrially late developers, due in part to their both being victims of imperial domination, Poland from the European and Russian powers and Greece from the Ottoman Empire. Now, however, the political, economic and social aspirations of both countries are focused much more towards the European Union, which has important implications for the countries health systems and professions of medicine and nursing. To the degree to which this is happening one can assert that 'convergence' is taking place (Saltman 1997). Political and policy reorientation within the health care system of a country does not, however, automatically lead to a complete adherence to the new regime. No reforms work on a clean slate – pre-existing social and cultural practices are typically strongly embedded (Granovetter 1992). These may be eventually erased and replaced by (or incorporated within) the new practices or they may co-exist with the new arrangements and continue to exert a strong influence. Mediterranean European countries, for instance, have all adapted national health systems in recent times (Katrougalos 1996), yet these are experienced very differently from the Liberal and Social

Democratic variants of Britain or Scandinavia. Despite organisational similarities to the Northern European versions, the histories and cultural expectations of the citizens as well as the professions are more akin to the State-Corporatist of France and Germany. As explained in Chapter 2 some observers view the welfare states of Greece, Italy, Spain and Portugal as underdeveloped versions of the corporatist model found in, for example, Germany and France (Katrougalos 1996:43). On another hand, it may be that this group of countries is more accurately viewed as a distinctive variety of welfare regime. Part of the quandary is whether the differences are explained best in terms of underdevelopment or different development.

Greece, while one of the Southern European countries (Ferrera 1996; Katrougalos 1996; Trifiletti 1999) is unlike the others in the group in not sharing the Latin/Catholic traditions and being Orthodox in its religion. Moreover, as Mouzelis (1986:xiii) points out, it shares a common history with the Balkans particularly in relation to their shared past under the rule of the Ottoman patrimonial empire with its intolerance of civil society which survived into the country's modern era. This was the outcome of a transition to parliamentary system of government without any strongly organised populist movements within the country (Mouzelis 1986:39).[1] It is this history that has left a particular clientelistic legacy on the political culture of the country. The differences with other European Mediterranean countries should not be overstated for Greece shares many social, cultural and political similarities with, for example, Italy and Spain (Katrougalas 1996).

East European governments of the ex-state socialist (that is, Communist) countries of Eastern Europe demonstrated great willingness – at least initially – to embrace free market solutions to the shortcomings in their welfare and health service provision. By the late 1990s, however, such solutions were found to be seriously flawed – not least because the citizens/consumers had no prior experience of dealing with such a system (Kokko, Hava, Ortun, and Leppo 1998:302). In the case of Poland, the Solidarity Government's strategy has been to implement a corporatist model both for health care delivery and professional organisation once the country had began to recover from the particularly bad economic situation of the 1980s and early 1990s, perhaps indicating that there was little commitment to the neo-liberal solutions on offer from the World Bank in the initial post-Communist era. Poland is an East European transitional society that has relatively recently emerged from Soviet control, it shares some similarity with the Mediterranean countries for it, too, culturally, has long been dominated by Catholic values. Also, post-Communist countries of Central Europe are in some senses 'underdeveloped' and in transition, although it was the Iron Curtain that shut Poland off from Europe rather than late development. Poland has a much larger population, at around 38.6 million (European Observatory – Poland 1999:1), than Greece which stood at 10.26 million in 1991 (European Observatory – Greece 1996:1) and has grown to nearer 10.4 million or more (Liaropoulos and Kaitelidou 1997:1). Greek citizens' life expectancy is one of the highest in the world (ibid.) while the Polish people suffer a life expectancy rather less than in Western Europe (the mortality rate rose during the 1970s and 1980s during the collapse of the Communist regime as it did in the rest of the region) (European Observatory – Poland 1999:2).

The chapter, in addition to exploring the issues of health care reforms and their implications for the medical and nursing professions, is particularly concerned with the issues of clientelism and familialism for reasons that will be made clear within the chapter. It is sufficient for the moment to state that clientelism (and to a lesser extent familialism) impinges directly on the policy and practice of health care in these two countries more than any other of the countries discussed here, including in all probability Italy. This is most apparent in the form of the 'little envelopes' that patients and/or their families expect to pay directly, but unofficially, to the doctors for their medical treatment. The argument that will be that such practices may well emerge when the health system is inadequate and/or the state is weak, but they may well be present for other socially and culturally embedded reasons too. This also ties in with the issue of nursing status and role within the health service, although it is more strongly tied to the question of 'familialism', the other half of the couplet that characterises patrimonial societies. The argument being made in this chapter is that medical malfeasance in Poland is more economically than culturally determined whereas in Greece, to an extent, the opposite is the case – even if economics plays an important part. There is an element of social embeddedness to the practice although this may well change as Greece becomes more integrated within the European Union. The same set of cultural expectations that legitimate medical clientelism in Greece also accounts for why nursing is generally held in low esteem. The chapter is divided into four parts followed by a conclusion. The first two parts are concerned with describing the health systems and the medical professions in both countries and the recent reforms being implemented. The third part deals not with clinical guidelines but also with another approach taken to ensure quality of care, the 'little brown envelopes' of extra illicit cash payments for medical treatment. This too, as with clinical quality systems, is analysed in terms of the implications for medical autonomy. Finally, and interrelatedly, the issue the relationship between nursing, familialism and gender is dealt with.

Healthcare reforms and hospital doctors

Poland

Poland's health expenditure as a percentage of its GDP stood at 6.2 in 1999 and of this the public sector accounted for 4.7 per cent (OECD 2000:9). The official figure is low compared to Western Europe, although it does become a little closer when one adds in an estimate for peoples' private expenditure, including the illicit 'little envelope' payments. The combined official and illicit figures raise health expenditure to around 6.7 per cent of GDP (the figure for 1994 cited in European Observatory – Poland 1999:19). In addition to the black economy there is also a small but legitimate private sector of primary and secondary care clinics. Some of the primary care clinics existed under the communist regime as 'physician co-operatives' (Duffy 1997:287, 310 fn. 15). Since 1989 there has also been a growth in private hospitals and in 1995 there were 27,000 officially recognised persons or companies engaged in private medical practice (Sobczak 1996:31).

The Polish people are very critical of their health services. Sobczak (1996:30–1) cites a 1995 opinion poll that reported 79 per cent of respondents considered the services as 'bad' or 'very bad'. In part, at least, this dissatisfaction reflects the antipathy people feel towards the need to pay 'more or less informal charges [co-payments] within the system of constitutionally guaranteed free health care services' (ibid.:31). Right from the beginning the post-1989 Solidarity governments developed plans for reforming the health organisation and financing of the health system which were set out in the 1991 Health Care Institutions Act (European Observatory – Poland 1999:49). The intention was (1) to introduce a quasi-market system to replace the command economy and (2) switch to an insurance-based (sickness fund) system. The reforms were dogged by the country's poor economic performance in the early 1990s (Sobczak 1998:7) with negative growth in 1991 and 1992 coupled with an alarming inflation rate of well over 500 per cent in 1990 (European Observatory – Poland 1999:3) which very seriously weakened what the Government could achieve and also undermined voters' confidence in the Solidarity Coalition Government too. This contributed to the election of a post-Communist coalition (known as the Democratic Left Alliance) between 1993 and 1998 which slowed down the quasi-market reforms politically (Duffy 1997:295). Whereas, the Solidaritys' (Centre – Right coalition) favoured a German health insurance model the Alliances' preferred reform options were more similar to the Swedish model with the emphasis on political decentralisation rather than hypothecation. The eventual reform implemented on 1 January 1999 was based on the German health insurance model but within a decentralised health delivery system.

The reform package implemented by the Solidarity-led coalition is one where the state guarantees a basic package of health services funded by a hypothecated system of sickness funds (Sobczak 1998:14–16). As in the German model the capital costs of public sector hospitals, clinics and related services are the responsibility of the regional states (*Voivodships*). These are administrative regions and not autonomous federal states, and central government reduced their number from 49 to 16 in 1999 on the grounds of administrative efficiency. It is this level of administration that has the responsibilty for the planning of the health services as well as for the regional hospitals and related services until, when and if these hospitals become self-managing institutions (European Observatory – Poland 1999:10–11). Until that time the regional specialist hospitals, along with the outpatient clinics and primary health care, will continue to be managed by the ZOZ (*Zespol Opieki Zdrowotnej*) health management units. These were established in 1972, originally as part of the central state control of health care based on the highly bureaucratic Soviet *Semashko* model that concentrated resources on the provision of acute, specialist hospitals (Kokko, *et al.* 1998:299–300). More recently the ZOZ have become the responsibility of the regional states but legislation has been passed allowing for ZOZ units to be dissolved (European Observatory – Poland 1999:10). However, it would appears that until a new system of local self-management is in place health care will remain under the management of the ZOZ units. Meanwhile, local government (*Powiats*) has been re-created and will become responsible for the district hospitals while primary health care is now increasingly the responsibility of the town and village councils, (*Gminas*). There are 2121 of these directly elected bodies, which along with local government are beginning to replace the ZOZ in the administration of the health services.

Central government retains overall control of very expensive and specialised services, notably organ transplants, as well as public health programmes. It is the Ministry of Health and Social Welfare that is responsible for policy and regulation of health care services and has oversight of medical schools, university hospitals and research institutes. Funding has been, since 1992, the responsibility of the Ministry of Finance. In addition, the ministries of defence, transport and those responsible for the prisons and police retain their own health services and manage their own health insurance fund. Together these ministries cover about 10 per cent of the workforce.

The financing of the country's health care is now provided by the 16 regional health insurance funds (that is, sickness funds), coterminous with the regional states (plus the additional fund for the armed and diplomatic services), as established under the 1997 Health Insurance Act (Kozierkiewicz and Karski 2001:34). This system is based on five principles: (1) universal participation; (2) contributions calculated on income (at 7.5 per cent); (3) 'social solidarity' ensuring equal access regardless of health risk; (4) self-governing health insurance funds; (5) the scheme guaranteed by the state (European Observatory – Poland 1999:49–50). Patients will normally have to pay an official co-payment for hospital bed and board as well as prescriptions charges for a wide range of drugs, medical materials and orthopaedic equipment (Sobczak 1998:14–16). The reforms officially came into force in January 1999; up until then the system was funded directly from government. Their introduction led to strikes within the medical profession (Reuters 1999) over real concerns that the reforms would lead to an increase in physician unemployment and a continued growth in private clinics (Duffy 1997:312, fn. 38), which has occurred (Kozierkiewicz and Karski 2001:35). The public's response to these reforms has also been lukewarm with more than 38 per cent of all patients less satisfied with the new arrangements than they were of the previous system (Czapinski and Panek 2000 cited in Kozierkiewicz and Karski 2001:35).

Hospital organisation

Hospital and outpatient services continue to reflect the hand of the Communist state that established the integrated but overbureaucratised services in the 1970s. Outpatient care is commonly provided by the policlinics as well as the primary care services. There was an attempt during the 1990s to replace this system with a system of general practice based around individual and group practices (European Observatory – Poland 1999:27; Sobczak 1996:15–16). Pilot schemes and training appear to have been successful but the model has yet to replace the pre-existing system of policlinics or, more importantly, overcome the low regard which primary care is held by health professionals and patients alike. The new family doctors are to be paid on a capitation basis by the *Voivodship* (regional state) or *Gmina* (directly elected town and village council). The next level in the system, in terms of acute services, is the 424 district general hospitals providing secondary care while more specialist care is provided by the 188 *Voivodship* hospitals. Then, at the regional and national level, there are the teaching hospitals that provide specialist tertiary care. Overall, the country has a low number of hospitals at 1.9 per 100,000 compared to the EU average of 3.8 in 1996 (European Observatory – Poland: 1999:32). If translated into hospital beds, figures show that only the UK has fewer beds per thousand population at 4.5 (European Observatory – UK 1999:76) compared with 5.19 for Poland (WHO 2001; OECD 2000).

Hospitals, whether they are the responsibility of a *Voivodship* or autonomous, are managed by a director who may be a manager or a physician. The director will report to a hospital executive board consisting of representatives of the staff, the trade unions and the *Gmina* (European Observatory – Poland 1999:30). Medical influence is largely through the management board which typically made up of heads of departments although the bureaucratic hand of ZOZ continued to exert influence throughout the 1990s and may still do so.

Greece

Health expenditure in Greece stands at 8.7 per cent of GDP (1999) (OECD 2002:8) of which spending on the public sector accounts for only 4.7 per cent, which is the lowest among the countries included here (ibid). The comparable figures for Poland are 6.2 and 4.6 per cent of GDP (OECD 2002:9). These total figures for both countries do not take into account the illicit informal payments to the doctors known in Greece as *fakelakia* (little envelopes) which may represent as much as a further 3 per cent of GDP paid directly to physicians (Kyriopoulas and Tsalikis 1993, cited in Liaropoulos and Kaitelidou 1997:3). This is a subject to be returned to later in the discussion of the Greek medical profession.

As with the other countries of the Mediterrranean Rim the Greek health service is based on a national health system, which is funded by a mix of sickness fund contributions and government funding. Sickness funds predate the Greek national health system (known as EΣY) and membership is based on occupation. The largest of the sickness funds is IKA, established in 1934 (European Observatory – Greece 1996:3), which covers industrial workers – manual and non-manual (OECD 1994:149). Rural workers (who make up over half the population) were without coverage until the setting up of the Agricultural Insurance Organisation (OGA) in 1961. Today, while there are around forty social health insurance organisations, the three largest cover 80 per cent of the population (ibid.:157). These are IKA, OGA and TEVE (small businesses and merchants). The range of health services covered varies between these organisations. All these funds will cover most aspects of hospital care[2] although not necessarily diagnostic and laboratory tests (OECD 1994:158; European Observatory – Greece 1996:19). These organisations are funded from employer and employee contributions except in the case of OGA, which the government funds entirely out of taxation. These funds cover just under one-third of the entire cost of the health care services (31.8 per cent in 1990) (OECD 1994:157) while general taxation contributes over a quarter of the revenue of the health service (26.3 per cent in 1990) (ibid.). The remaining just over 40 per cent is an estimation of private payments (Sissouras, Karokis and Mossialos 1999:365). This overlaps extensively with the widespread 'underground economy of health' (Colombotos and Fakiolas 1993:140).

The health service, EΣY, was introduced by the Greek Socialist Party (PASOK) after it came to power in 1981, the legislation being passed in 1983.[3] These reforms were based on five principles (European Observatory – Greece 1996:5):

1 universal coverage and equal access with the state responsible for overall provision
2 a primary health care based system 'gatekeeping' access to specialist and hospital care
3 primary and secondary health care to be provided by public sector facilities and private hospitals to be prohibited
4 a decentralised system with health councils established in the regions providing planning and administration co-ordinated nationally by the Central Health Council (KEΣY); membership to include representatives of the insurance funds, providers, trade unions and medical schools as well as the Ministry of Health
5 health care professionals, including doctors, to be wholly employed by EΣY and paid a salary.

During the 1980s the government increased public health expenditure to around 5 per cent, increased doctors salaries substantially, and planned to build 18 new hospitals, including three regional university hospitals, as well as 400 health centres across the country. There would also be closer integration between the Government and the insurance funds. The reality was less impressive. The three university hospitals were built (Ioannina, Patras and Crete) and a large number of private clinics were closed down resulting in a reduction of the number of hospitals overall. Private diagnostic centres were allowed because the cost of the technology was prohibitive for the health service to provide from within ΕΣΥ itself. Even so the cost of the services provided were themselves a significant burden.

Primary care health centres in the rural areas were implemented but staffed mostly by inexperienced doctors, and the system never provided a referral service for the hospitals. No primary care centres were ever established in urban areas as this would have encroached on the IKA health services, which had been set up in the 1930s and provided a relatively comprehensive service, although user satisfaction is generally low (Matsaganis 1998:342). There were three other disappointments for the supporters of ΕΣΥ. These were, first, the continuing high levels of private practice by many, possibly most, ΕΣΥ doctors despite the doubling of doctors' salaries during this period and its official prohibition. The practice was and continues to be universally tolerated. Second, the integration between the sickness funds and government was very limited and in effect has led to the Ministry of Health subsidising the sickness funds by setting the premium levels of the members and the fees to the providers so that by the early 1990 the state was paying 88 per cent of health care costs directly (ibid.: 6). At the same time the sickness funds have kept their separate identities and IKA continues to provide the health centre services in the urban areas and effectively runs a parallel health service. Third, decentralisation never happened and the regional health councils have never materialised.

In 1992 the then Conservative Government amended the 1983 legislation to allow greater flexibility, possibly reflecting more the reality of the Greek society and public life. Certainly this was the case with allowing doctors to choose to between full- or part-time contracts with ΕΣΥ and in the latter case permitting some private practice. Equally, emphasising patients' freedom of choice simply endorsed what was happening anyway, a reason why the primary care referral system never worked. This Conservative Government also permitted private for-profit hospitals to operate but it was too short-lived to be able to implement its programme.

On returning to power PASOK rescinded the 1992 legislation and set up two committees to advise it on how best to reform the health system: the local committee of Greek experts to advise it on the organisation and management of the system, and the international committee (Abel-Smith *et al.* 1994) whose recommendations were for the most part incorporated into the subsequent reform legislation. The key elements of the report were as follows:

1   public sector hospitals to become autonomous entities within public ownership, similar to 'trust' hospitals within the UK
2   hospital doctors to be paid on a retrospective 'fee for service' points scheme similar to the German model for ambulatory care (see Knox 1993:88; Busse and Howorth 1999:308); private practice to be abolished or restricted to senior doctors only
3   sickness funds and government contributions to be pooled within one unified fund
4   the reformed health system to be based on a family doctor service, very similar to general practice in the UK, including management of their own budgets; these doctors to be paid on a capitation basis designed to ensure an equivalent income to that of hospital specialists.

In the event the 'ambivalence of the political authorities' (Sissouras *et al.* 1999:391) and the social and cultural realities ensured the eventual policies were substantially diluted. It is now very unlikely that the largest sickness funds will lose their identity by becoming integrated into the unified health insurance fund. IKA will also take on the responsibility for establishing the GP network within the urban areas, reinforcing its established role as the main provider of primary care services. On the other hand, the emphasis on decentralisation set out in the original 1983 legislation did gain support, with new legislation in 1997 setting out a policy for the EΣY to be managed by regional health authorities (but within more of a purchaser – provider framework) and there is some indication of a commitment to switch from per diem charges to global budgets leading on to a more detailed DRG-like based system of accounting for hospitals (Sissouras *et al.* 1999:392). There is also an emphasis on health promotions and prevention as well as quality of care and quality assurance issues, although here the main concern is health technology assessment, a response to the high cost the EΣY, and sickness funds have paid over the 1980s and 1990s for an uncontrolled expansion of medical high technology such as CAT scans (Matsaganis 1998:340).

Whether reforms will take root will depend on wider political considerations and the implications these have at the local level. The current political debate is largely around the question of European integration (Petmesidou 1996:340–4) and there would appear to be some content to this debate with the implication that, eventually, state clientelism might be replaced by greater administrative rationality. In the 1999 spring PASOK party congress, for example, the country's premier, Costas Simitis, argued strongly for EMU (European Monetary Union) remaining the government's primary goal on the grounds that it will change the economic, social and cultural map of Greece (*Athens News* 1999:3). There are parallels here with the Polish case, although less to do with party political clientelism (which has more in common with Italy's *partitocrazia*) than with the two countries both being in a process of transition – along different routes perhaps but both have set a course from the European periphery towards the centre of the European Union. To achieve this, among other things the two countries have to establish a system of governance that rationalises their welfare regimes along certain lines compatible with the current members of the European Union. This includes the organisation and practices of the health professions, which brings me to the issue of the medical professions in these two countries and the question as to whether similar practices reflect similar causes or not. This has a bearing on the broader question of isomorphism or convergence between health care systems.

Poland

Hospital doctors and the 'gift' relationship

Hospital doctors and the medical profession generally are very low paid compared to Western standards. They earn, officially, less than an industrial worker. An anaesthetist at a Warsaw hospital, in May 1998, told me 'Now we have basic salary it is about 1,000 zloty for the doctor...per month. Altogether with their duty etcetera, it is over 2,000 [*zloty*] which in Euros equates to around €560 or £370 a month. Even by Polish standards this is a low figure. In 1993, for example, doctors' pay was about 86 per cent of the average for Poland, which was low in any case having fallen to 71 per cent of the 1989 figure and only rising to about 78 per cent in 1996 (European Observatory – Poland 1999:35). It is perhaps surprising that the post-Communist regimes would be continuing the Communist tradition of treating expert labour (*intelligentsia*) as socially inferior to the blue-collar workers in terms of pay. Duffy (1997:309, fn. 7), for example, reports that in 1975 health care workers earned 22 per cent less than industrial workers and the 'discrepancy widened in subsequent years'. At the same time the profession enjoys high social prestige, which in part reflects the religious culture of the country; medicine was a vocation close to the priesthood. However, not all physicians behaved as saints.

Pre-1989 hospital physicians, to boost their income, would often leave work early to see private patients, sometimes taking medical supplies and medication with them (ibid:287). The same practice continues today. Working in private clinics after the end of their day's work in the public sector (3.00 p.m.) is not uncommon and is often viewed as a financial necessity, as the following comment from one of the doctors quoted earlier illustrates: 'I am a leading...[specialist] in my country... I am not living in such a fancy place, I have a normal flat...and *still* I have to go three times a week to the...private practice...to just to make my living! This is totally crazy!' The other common practice among many physicians is the routine expectation of illicit co-payments ('little envelopes') from their patients, a practice that is estimated to double their salary (European Observatory – Poland 1999:17–18). As in Greece, this practice is neither legitimate nor penalised. Doctors are not disciplined, dismissed or taken to court for the malpractice. These payments are 'required' for referring patients to specialists and for operations. For a major operation this will be around one year's salary. According to research by the Sociological Analysis Group[4] at the Centre of Health System Management (Warsaw) the practice has been becoming more widespread in the post-Communist era. In 1992, 16 per cent of their sample reported having made payments; the figure in 1998 had risen to 29 per cent[5] (see also Chawla *et al.* 1998; European Observatory – Poland 1999:17). These 'little envelopes' are in reality not that small; moreover, if the patient does not go along with the system then she or he does not get treatment. One hospital doctor from Warsaw (May 1998) explained how the system worked.

> you go to the private office of the Chief of the Department. And you pay him for admi[tting] you to the hospital...this [is a] well known price, so he admits you to his own Department...And then, there is a problem of operation! Yeah? So they propose...for example, [an] operation is needed to cure your problem...So, you have to pay [more] money...For your own doctor on the ward, not for the Chief... but, it depends on...circumstances. And then, the operation is done.

In the case of an acute admission the situation is transformed from informal private practice to something altogether darker, as this doctor explained.

> If you have for example, brain tumour, [an] acute illness...you are admitted...as acute case to oncology clinic. So you *have* to pay, your

family has to pay, has to pay *before* operation! Because otherwise they...don't *do* [the] operation...[because] you are not good for anaesthesia, we have not time, we have no doctors!

Patients requiring surgery can expect to have to pay out the equivalent of a little over one years salary, 50 per cent has to be paid before and 50 per cent after. An academic I arranged to meet to discuss Polish heath policy turned out to have been very ill with a brain tumour. He recounted his and his family's experience of the functioning of the informal health economy in brain surgery without a note of rancour.

> Some people advised my family to try to get treatment abroad. But they said the doctors are so qualified [and] of such high quality there is no need to go abroad...it w[ould also] cost a huge amount of money, so it [wa]s out of question, to go to the private hospital. I stayed at the [public] hospital for three and half months so it would [have] be[en] disastrous I ha[d] no...private health insurance so I would have [had] to pay out of my salary...[U]niversity salaries [are] even lower than doctors salaries.

His family was never asked for the 'little envelope' payments but they knew it was expected of them and they knew too that if they did not pay he would not have the operation. It was a matter discussed within the family and among close friends. The payment made amounted to a little more than his annual salary. He was treated at a large public hospital in Warsaw where he believed he was well looked after.

The doctors take the 'little envelopes' according to the hospital doctor quoted earlier:

> [first,] because you are very, very, bad[ly] paid, by Government, so...you have family and so on and so on and so on. So you take this money...and the second [reason] is...you are involved in the whole system in the clinic. As a young doctor you come to the...clinic, and you try...to be independent...[but] you can't be independent, because they all take money...So you have to be involved in the group of people taking money. If not, you are [to be] excluded! So you *have* to...be paid.

The practice of giving the 'little envelopes' has been rationalised on the grounds that it is a long-standing tradition for patients or their families presenting a gift to the physician following satisfactory treatment

(Duffy 1997:311, fn. 22) although the practice in its current form evolved under the Communist regime and was commonplace by the end of the 1970s as a response to the inadequacies and shortages of the system (European Observatory – Poland 1999:17). The private payment was made in the expectation that the patient would get quicker and better treatment than would otherwise be the case. The practice continued after the collapse of the Communist regime and remains strongly embedded within the health care system, although the hope of the policy makers is that the new system of health insurance will eradicate this corrupt practice (Sobczak 1996:31) and will formalise the relations between public and private. Any success in this will depend in part on sufficient economic growth to fund the changes and ensure that a shift in the expectations of the doctors can and does take place.

Alongside the 'little envelopes' are other practices which doctors employ to help patients cope with the official cost of their treatment, at least in relation to the cost of drugs. One doctor already quoted outlined three methods employed in order to access expensive drugs more cheaply for patients.

> [First method] we do this clinical trial...and we have very, very good prices for, for the drug...The second method is, we can [help] parents...for example, apply [to] a foundation or...companies to have money...for a very, very expensive treatment...or we [put] some...notes [that is advertisements] in newspapers that we collect money for example...for a transplantation. And the third method is not so official! [W]e can buy some drugs on 'Green [prescription form]', [which]...is a receipt [that is, prescription form] – paid 100 per cent...refunded by Government...this is...a 'small door' for us...because this is not precisely...defined...and we try to...go through this 'door'...we write this Green receipts...for patients.

Clearly, much of medical practice – as well as payments – are carried out outside not only of the official health care system but beyond the remit of the organised profession too. These practices raise fundamental questions as to whether professions are themselves a legitimated form of clientelism, with a responsibility of advising patients how best to negotiate the complexities of health care or, as in the case of Poland and Greece, licensed to practice as a means of institutionalising the subterranean economy of health care not amenable to government regulation. Western governments prefer the first to be the case, with its connotation of 'responsible autonomy'.

The medical profession

The Polish medical profession was originally formally constituted in 1921 with the establishment of the doctors' chambers – or medical councils (*Izba Lekarska*). by the Polish parliament (*Sejm*). This was an autonomous self-governing organisation responsible for the registration of physicians and their right to practice (Kennedy and Sadkowski 1991:186). There was a medical council for each province (*voivodship*) and a central council that negotiated with government, similar to the German model. Under Communist rule all pre-existing professional organisations, including the doctors' chambers, were disbanded and the work of physicians was placed under the direct control of the Ministry of Health and Social Welfare. Under the Communist regime, however, new collective organisations for doctors along with other health care workers were introduced. In 1946 the Trade Union of Health Workers' Party (*Polska Zjednoczona Partia Robotnicza* – PZPR) was established (Kennedy and Sadowsky 1991:186) and in 1952 the Polish Physicians' Association (*Polskie Towarzystwo Lekarskie*) was founded as a scientific association. This latter organisation still functions today and, according to the physicians I spoke with, is generally well thought of within the profession, as the following quote from the anaesthetist cited earlier shows:

> [The scientific associations] exist for a long time, and...prescribed a level for education for each surgeon [that is doctor] in Poland...[I]t was an independent association and...the[e] rules [that is advice] was accepted by Minister of Health [under Communist regime]. Minister didn't control, Minister *only* accepts!...Now it is accepted by Medical Chamber and [the] Minister.

The profession, however, did not regain any real autonomy until the rise of Solidarity and the establishment of its Medical Sections (ibid. 1991:185). These medical sections include nurses, ambulance drivers, porters and other health care workers as well as physicians. What holds this disparate collection of occupations together is the very success of the Solidarity movement. There are other independent trade unions for physicians and possibly the most important is the Trade Union of Polish Physicians (*Zwiazek Zawodowy Lekarzy Polskich*: ZZLP). During the 1980s it had around 9000 members or 12 per cent of physicians. By contrast it has been estimated that about 90 per cent of physicians were members of the Medical Sections of Solidarity with

20 per cent being activists (ibid. 1991:188). The Medical Sections are still influential and remain the main forum for health workers expression of autonomy.

The other major change for the medical profession has been the recreation of the specifically professional body, the Doctors' Chamber (*Izba Lekarska*), which might be seen as antagonistic to the role of the Medical Sections and it certainly would appear to be the case that some physicians, particularly those from the medical schools, did seek to establish independent professional control of their own specific occupation and its organisation. The Polish Physicians' Association (*Polskie Towarzystwo Lekarskie*) submitted proposals for the resurrection of *Izba Lekarska* to the *Sejm* (Parliamentary) Commission on Health Care in 1983 but it was not re-established until 1989 (Duffy 1997:299; European Observatory – Poland 1999:50). This body is of a different order of self-organisation from the Solidarity model, for it is not a union but has much more in common with the German *Ärztekammer* with responsibility for licensing practitioners and conditions of clinical practice as well as postgraduate education and training. It also has the responsibility of maintaining standards within the profession (for example, inspection and licensing of private clinics). The chamber, however, has not been universally welcomed from within the profession, being viewed as an instrument of elite domination by senior academic professors. As one hospital specialist commented, 'they [a]re chosen by, names, positions, probably connections, but not by...democracy'. Nevertheless, the reintroduction of the Doctors' Chambers does mean that the institutional arrangements for an autonomous medical profession are now in place within Poland: scientific associations, unions and the Doctors' Chambers. This model shares much with the German system reflecting Poland's particular *Mitteleuropean* institutional history and provides the organised profession with considerable formal autonomy from the state. Whether this will also mean the profession will be able to drive out unprofessional practices such as the 'little envelopes' remains to be seen, although this may be more connected to economic growth and dependent upon greater investment in health care than professional integrity on its own.

Quality of medical care

Evidence-based medicine and clinical guidelines appear not to have made much impact on the delivery of medical care as yet. There is currently a programme of accreditation underway instigated by the Ministry of Health and Social Welfare who, in the late 1990s, commissioned the Association of Hospitals and the Chamber of Physicians to define the standards to be implemented by the National Hospital Accreditation Committee (European Observatory – Poland 1999:32). Two other bodies centrally involved in this work are the Health Services Quality Assessment Centre in Krakow and the National Centre for Health System Management from Warsaw. It is too early to state with any certainty the outcome of this process but there is little doubt that accreditation will be associated with a radical restructuring of the hospitals system (ibid) and possibly the loss of medical posts. In this context it is likely that the hospital doctors will resent any adoption of clinical guidelines and related practices as a top-down imposition that will be associated with a general rationalisation of the hospital services and increasing unemployment for hospital doctors too.

The one area where clinical guidelines are likely to be more readily adopted will be associated with drug trials funded by pharmaceutical companies. This is a useful source of additional resources as the Polish paediatrician quoted earlier has pointed out.

Greece

The medical profession

The Greek state is technically responsible for determining the numbers of physicians trained. Moreover, there are only a limited number of places at the seven medical schools within the country. It might therefore seem strange that Greece is provided with an excessive number of hospital specialists (the opposite is true of the primary care clinics). There are 3.9 doctors per 1000 in Greece compared with 2.4 per 1000 in Poland (WHO – 2002). There are more doctors per head of population[6] than in most other countries in Europe *except* Spain and Italy (European Observatory – Greece 1996:47). The fact is that many would-be doctors enrol at a medical school abroad mostly in Italy where the universities are far less restricted in the numbers of medical students they can recruit. Others will study in Eastern European countries. Having got their medical degree the aspiring Greek physicians need only undertake a practical examination in order to become licensed. They may not find employment in the public sector and in any case they will have to wait for a while before a post becomes available, for graduates are required to register on Ministry of Health waiting lists according to their intended area of specialisation.

Hospital organisation

Within each hospital there is a scientific committee, which is a legally established body that functions very much as a medical staff committee. While certainly not all, many doctors are critical of its perceived lack of effectiveness, as illustrated by an oncology specialist from Athens interviewed in September 1998: 'Nobody *listens* to this Committee because the President, the Board of Directors in the hospital are...entirely from the [Government] Ministry! They do what the Ministry thinks correct! Not the Scientific Committee.'

Since 1997 the work of doctors within hospitals has become the responsibility of the medical director similar to the situation in Italy – and elsewhere, although the effectiveness of the person in post appears to be measured more according to clientelistic criteria than any other, as one doctor explained: 'It depends on the person, it's always happens in Greece, it depends on the person.' A characteristic also of the country's organised medical profession too.

Professional organisations

Greek medical organisation reflects the French and Italian model. There are three types of collective medical organisations: (1) official medical societies; (2) specialist medical societies; (3) physicians' unions. Each has peculiarities of its own.

Official medical societies

The Pan Hellenic Medical Society (*Panellionios Iatrikos Sillogos – PIS*) was established in 1923 and codified in 1939 under the Metaxas dictatorship (Colombotos and Fakiolas 1993:141). Membership of one of the 58 local societies is mandatory. While appearing to have similarities to the Doctor's Chambers in Poland the fact that it was imposed from above rather than demanded by, at least, a part of the profession does make an important difference even if (1) the Polish 'Chambers' were demanded by the profession's elite only and (2) the basic roles performed by both institutions are very similar. The local medical societies in Greece have the responsibility for the detailed administration of the profession within their areas including disciplinary procedures. The organisation, however, is generally seen as having limited influence even over key professional issues including education, training and professional development (ibid.:142), for it is designed more as an instrument of state control (even if an ineffective one) than it is one of self-management and professional autonomy.

Specialist medical societies

As elsewhere in Europe there is a wide range of learned societies. Unlike their Polish equivalents, however, their influence within the profession is very limited because, similar to the situation in Italy, the state pays little attention to the work of these bodies (ibid.:143). This, however, can be overstated for they are the only reasonably autonomous organisational space the profession has for discussing clinical developments and medical science. Moreover, they provide a useful informal network for academic physicians who are commonly believed to have an important influence on government's appointments within the health sector and on related policy. There is also some evidence that these societies are growing in influence, again similar to the Italian situation. To quote a medical chief of an Athens Hospital interviewed in September 1998:

> Just now they [Ministry of Health is] starting to approve some kind of participation of the Societies to specialties, training, certification and all that stuff. Just this summer we have proposed to the Ministry where we could contribute. There is a tendency, in the context of the EC, for the medical associations to be part of the system...At the moment they're trying to broaden...and give some kind of authority to the medical associations...It's only minor. Just a little. Actually it works a little politically...for example, the Minister has some counsellors around him, most of them are chosen among his friends, and his friends are chosen among the political party that comes to power...So, all the societies are successful, depending on how many members of their, are close to the Ministry of Health.

All of which sounds very similar to the French situation in that the political culture ignores the notion of 'subsidiarity' in favour of *étatisme* and would be legitimated by reference to the Rousseaunian principle of the 'general will', for it was part of the ideology of Greek independence (Mouzelis 1986: 41), but in the Greek context rather than *étatisme* the result is rule through clientelistic networks. It is against this background that one can begin to understand reasons behind the more recent emergence of doctors' unions.

Physicians' unions

More active in providing an independent voice for the physicians are the physicians' unions. The best known, and largest, of these is the Union of Hospital Physicians or EINAP (*Enosis Iatron Nosileftirion,*

Athinon-Piraeus), which was established in 1976 and represents around 8000 salaried physicians (Colombotos and Fakiolas 1993). The second largest is the Society of Professional Health Personnel of IKA, or SEIPIKA (*Sillogos Epistimonikou Igionomikou Prosopikou*, IKA), which represented around 6000 physicians (ibid). There are regional counterparts throughout Greece of both organisations which are linked together with EINAP and SEIPIKA within a federation. Their support comes from the doctors' desire to defend their interests and therefore unsurprisingly these organisations too are marked with the imprint of clientelism, with EINAP having PASOK (Pan Hellenic Socialist Party) representatives sitting on its central committees (Colombotos and Fakiolas 1993:143).

Medical professionalism

Clientelism has particular implications for medical ethics and doctor – patient relations, for good practice does not appear to be recognised as the universal duty by doctors but is, instead, an obligation only to those patients who have sought out the services of a specific physician and have paid an 'honorarium' or 'little envelope' (known in Greece as *fakelakia*). This may possibly be a function of low pay, but even though this may play a part it is not the whole reason, as will be explained.

The simplest way to understand the phenomena is that it is inversely related to the physicians' low salaries which reflect the poor economic performance of the country generally. The Greek health system has suffered from the country's low economic growth ('close to zero') in the 1980s and early 1990s (Petmesidou 1996:326). Although paralleling Poland in some respects the country never suffered anything like the negative growth experienced by Poland during the same period. As for the doctors, in 1992 their EΣY salary was between $9500 and $19,000 (US) (that is, approximately £6000 to £12,000) while that of the IKA physicians was even lower (Colombotos and Fakiolas 1993:140). At the same time, private practice and *fakelakia* earnings averaged a little over $30,000 (US), that is, very approximately £19,000) (ibid.:139). Informal payments are virtually universal in the case of surgery and professors command the highest fees of all. There is little attempt by the authorities to curb or stop these activities. One probable reason is that, unlike their Polish counterparts, middle-class families would worry even more if the were not able to pay 'out of pocket' to ensure a good service from the physician. Patients often distrust public health care services and will commonly seek second opinions, third and more opinions, and this partly explains the general belief that paying for a physician ensures better-quality treatment (OECD 1994:153). As one surgeon

I met in March 1999 explained, this is a process by which patients can ensure they get the personal attention of the specialist, generally a better quality of service, and are able to 'jump the queue' (see also European Observatory – Greece 1996:21):

> [T]here is a relationship between the surgeon and the patient... particularly for morally obligated cases...I use every Saturday to spend...two or three hours and this is the time that I have... see friends...who work here. They come to find me and to ask me to see one friend...unofficially.

I asked whether he was paid for this service; he replied:

> This is a problem...I think that the hospital loses some money from this...because...one third of the patients that I see is unofficial... I examine, and on Monday I give his name to the secretary...To the [operating] list...sometimes in front of the others.

Note how the arrangements are discussed in terms of obligations between friends and are driven by more than (black or grey) market economics; rather they are a correlate of the clientelistic culture of Greek public life. Perversely, *fakelakia* transactions are socially embedded, culturally rationalised and seem to be universally accepted, yet they are formally illegal. They reflect a most unusual form of 'loose-coupling'. The most recent WHO report for Greece (European Observatory – Greece 1996:58) states that, following the introduction of the EΣΥ in 1983 doctors received fairly high salaries and this was reflected in some reduction in the unofficial payments. Today doctors received about twice the average for public employment but this is much lower in relative terms than their earnings in 1983. Over the same time there has been a growth in unofficial payments so that now they are estimated to increase a doctor's income by approximately 40 per cent on average (ibid). Sissouras, Karokis and Mossialos (1994:152) cite research that indicates that the informal economy amounts to just over half of the total health expenditure, which corresponds with Liaropoulos and Tragakes's (1998:159–60) estimate based on 1992 figures that it amounts to 3.43 per cent of GDP. This translates to families spending an estimated 25 per cent of the cost of health care in out-of-pocket cash payments (Colombotus and Fakiolas 1993:139).

The Greek citizen, similarly to their Polish counterpart, is commonly dissatisfied with the health service. Collectively they are one of the most dissatisfied in the Europe Union along with Italy and Portugal (Mossialos 1997:111). Over half (53.9 per cent) of Greeks were either 'fairly' or 'very' dissatisfied with their health system while the figure for Italy was 59.4 per cent and Portugal 59.3 per cent. In part, patients' suspicions as to the quality of health service provision may be well founded. As an illustration, a Greek newspaper, *ELEFTHEROTYPIA* (*Freepress* 1999:16), reported that there was a 'Third World situation in 59 major Greek hospitals', at least according to the Consumer Council in Greece. Nevertheless, the patients' own approach to health care services exacerbates the inequalities and the quality of care. The culture of clientelism supports an individualistic and familial culture with value being placed on particularistic/discretionary health care provision (and welfare generally). This creates the ambivalent attitude and approach to the health system and the physicians. This is why seeking out a good physician involves getting several opinions. In these terms *fakelakia* is a characteristic of how clientelistic relations are sustained rather than, primarily, a function of low medical salaries.

Résumé

In Greece and Poland there is a long tradition of unofficial, informal but widely accepted practice of illicit co-payments. This is a means by which many middle-class patients and their families (1) exercise choice, (2) gain access to scarce resources and (3) compensate physicians for their relative low levels of pay (Kutzin 1998:93; Abel-Smith *et al.* 1994). This practice puts a different gloss on the notion of medical autonomy. Rather than being 'de-coupled' (Meyer and Rowan 1991) from the formal structures of the organisation in order to deliver health care services more effectively the autonomy the doctors enjoy is 'uncoupled', separated from, the formal organisation in the sense that the informal payments, queue jumping and misappropriating hospital materials undermine the organisation effectiveness. 'Uncoupled' autonomy (Figure 6.1) reflects a situation when the work of the individual medical practitioners is not compatible with that of the interests of the state or the organised profession. Greek society is currently subject to pressures of 'disembedding' (Giddens 1991:209) and 're-embedding' within a Western European and more global mode, which if successful will take the regime a long way from its roots in the specificities of patrimonial social and political relations. Current political debates in Greece and its governing party (PASOK) are precisely around these notions. Poland, I would suggest, is different and despite parallels of being a late developer on the periphery of Europe there is less cultural space for 'uncoupled'

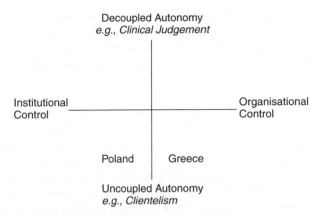

Figure 6.1   Uncoupled autonomy and professionalism

autonomy of the medical profession (or any other group) to survive in the longer run and if the health reforms take hold and the Doctors' Chamber can establish their authority within the profession then one can expect the system of illicit payments to be squeezed out of the system. Whereas Greece has a history that can culturally legitimate *fakelakia*, Poland does not; rather it is a *Rechtsstaat* state that has had a long sojourn under Soviet hegemony. The practice of illicit 'little envelopes', in its modern form, acts as an illicit gatekeeper to medical services rather than as in Greece where it is more a means of improving the quality of care. These 'little envelopes' are less culturally embedded in Poland than in Greece even if they are widely tolerated.

In the case of nursing the issues of social embeddedness is also a crucial dimension but here the dynamics relate much more to the influence of familialism and its ability to restrict the autonomy and status of the profession rather than 'uncouple' it as is the case with doctors.

Nursing: gender, familialism and clientelism

This section examines the variations in the professional and gendered organisation of nursing in Greece and Poland. The argument presented here will be that the gendered nature of nursing is embedded within broader social as well as work relations, including familialism and clientelism. Nursing in both Poland and Greece is predominantly female, low paid, and not a popular choice of career in as much as there are nursing shortages in both countries. In Poland, the public generally holds the occupation in high regard while in Greece it does not. Yet in both countries nursing, historically, was imbued with a degree of religious vocationalism that stemmed from its links with the Church: Catholic in the case of Poland, Orthodox in the case of Greece.

Poland

Under the state socialist regime nurses lost their professional status in the 1960s and no longer have a voice in the Ministry of Health (Brykczynska 1992:21) despite a long tradition of professional organisation starting with the training of ecclesiastical and lay nuns at Lvov in 1895 and the establishment of a modern nursing school in Krakow in 1911 (Stecka-Feffer 1996:72). The Polish Association of Professional Nursing (PSPZ) was created in 1923, a University Department of Nurses and Hygienists was opened in Krakow in 1925, and the profession gained legal recognition in 1936. In the post-Communist period after 1989 the nursing profession has regained its formal status and it now has its own 'chamber' responsible for nurse registration, standards and ethics.

Nurse education is also in the process of change. While there has been a graduate nurse programme since the 1970s (Brykczynska 1992:21) the majority of nurses have entered the profession via a five-year nurses training programme starting at around fifteen years of age (ibid.: 22). This approach is now seen as inappropriate and inflexible and the five-year programme has been phased out in favour of a three-year diploma, which does not recruit students until after they have completed secondary education, unlike previously (European Observatory – Poland 1999:39).

At a different level altogether to this basic nurse education, academic nursing courses are well established even if they are a minority activity. There are several centres attached to universities where nurses can undertake degree studies in nursing sciences, and the figures of the early 1990s indicate that slightly over 1 per cent of nurses had a degree. These nurses were primarily employed in teaching and administration. In 1998 there were two nurses with PhDs completing their 'habilitation'[7] with the intention of becoming professors, one at Lublin, the other at Cracow.

Continuing education and training, by contrast, is fairly haphazard and is largely carried out by physicians for their clinical areas. The authors of the European Observatory – Poland (1999:40) report: '[Nurses] mostly remain subordinate to doctors in the practice of their work... [and] carry less responsibility than nurses in most western European health systems...undertak[ing] tasks that in cost-effective terms should be performed by support staff'.

Polish nurses are caught in a double bind. Their work was officially viewed as secondary to that of direct labour of the 'proletariat' under communism (this was also true of the medical profession), and while the state ideology has changed the pay differential has not. In 1999 the *Guardian* (10 July:17), reporting a nurses' hunger strike, quoted the average monthly wage as being £65. At the same time, being gendered female, particularly within this strongly Catholic country, meant these women are viewed principally as 'wives and mothers' rather than 'workers' (see Trifiletti 1999). The situation has strong similarities with other Eastern European countries and the following description of the relationship between family and work under Communism in the Czech Republic could equally describe the situation in Poland.

> The criterion for personal prestige...became tied to one's family image. The family turned into the dominant social institution, to the extent that we can almost consider it a public institution. There was also a counter-effect to this tendency. While the family remained the last bastion of freedom, the workplace remained the last gathering place outside the family. Both private and public problems were discussed at work, and often work time was partially devoted to arranging private matters. (Havelková 1993:92)

This situation did not disappear with the 'Velvet Revolution'. While freedom of speech is real enough, so is the lack of freedom from economic and financial stringency, and it is this that ensures the family remains a key institution. With the family comes a wider network of contacts, loyalties and obligations. This situation, however, is more the result of the inadequacy of the public services than with any official/state commitment to subsidiarity – despite the influence of the Catholic Church. In practice, the family functions, at least among the professional and managerial strata, to provide support for individual members. There are, again, parallels here with Greece.

Greece

Modern nurse training in Greece dates from 1875 under royal patronage, followed shortly after by the establishment of a nursing school at the Evangelismos Hospital in 1881. During this same period the Hellenic Red Cross was offering short nursing courses for volunteer nurses although they were not to offer a two-year programme, organised on the UK model, until 1914 (Quinn and Russell 1993:100). The point being made here is that the Nightingale model of hospital nursing influenced Greek nursing development from an early period and, as it happens, earlier than most Continental or Southern European countries (for example, France, Germany and Italy). This early development, however, has not prevented the public failing to recognise the professional status of nursing in Greece. Today Greek nurse education and training is similar to that found across Europe, with general nurses receiving a three-year 'technological nursing education' leading to a nursing diploma. This system was introduced in the 1980s. Nursing students are taught at the technological educational institutions. There are also training courses for assistant nurses of two years duration provide at the vocational nursing schools attached to hospitals (ibid.: 47). Selection for one of these courses is by the national system of Pan-Hellenic examinations, which operates as a general 'sorting office' for college and university courses as well as professional training (Lanara 1996:41). There are also one-year specialisation courses in clinical nursing and other similar courses for nurse teacher training and nurse management for the qualified nurse.

As in Poland, and much of the rest of Europe too, there is a shortage of nurses, but as a senior nurse explained in September 1998:

> everybody has realised, [including] the Minister of Health...that we need the nurses in the hospitals...We have very few!...*But*, this is not a good time...because of the economic situation, and the European Community, ECUs and all these things...So, it's not easy for [government] to give money...they only economise...[F]or example, ten nurses retiring, and we hire five! So...of course...we can't increase the well-educated nurses at the hospitals. It could take many years!

There is a nursing department at the University of Athens, founded in 1979. Two more are planned, one at the University of Crete the other at Thráki in Northern Greece. The nursing department in Athens has provided a nursing degree programme since 1987 and graduate programmes since 1993. The first PhD in Nursing was awarded in 1987. Despite the formal emphasis on qualifications and educational status of nursing, in Greece it has low status. This is partly because a nursing career probably means the person failed to achieve what they really hoped for in the national examinations and because the Greek health service is limited in its resources. But, the more fundamental (socially embedded) reason is because the giving of care is the family's responsibility – not the state's or its nursing employees'. This is an overstatement of the situation, but it is not incorrect. When the family members cannot be with the patient (as during the night) they will, if they can afford it, hire private nurses to sit with the patient. This is partly because they do not trust the nursing staff to provide good care, but it is reflects the familial and clientelistic character of Greek society.

Conclusions

The modern history of the Polish and Greek health care systems and the organised medical profession in these countries reflects a complex set of relations between the physicians, their patients and the state. Here Granovetter's (1992) discussion of embeddedness, trust and malfeasance in economic life (see also Geertz's study of the north African bazaar economy) this helps to explain the variations in the systems of illicit co-payments between Poland and Greece. And the basis of this variation is the differences in their embeddedness and the relationship this has to trust and malfeasance in medical care. Both Polish and Greek societies have relied on familialism and clientelism to compensate for the deficit of stateness. Moreover, policy makers in both countries believe that by adopting Western European solutions to the problems of health care provision they will be able to drive out the illicit practices. What is less clear is whether such policies would also change the people's perception of nursing.

The feminised character of nursing is not simply a consequence of the doctor–nurse division of labour and boundaries; it is also shaped by its relations with familialism within the configuration of health care services. The sexual division of labour in relation to care giving within the paid labour force cannot be divorced from that within the family (O'Connor 1996:17). This is not only related to the over-representation of women within this predominantly low-wage type of work; it also relates to the embedded cultural values associated with it and – in the case of nursing – this does vary systematically according to welfare regime type. Familialism also relates to the clientelistic relations that pervade health care delivery (and welfare provision generally) in both countries (Petmesidou 1996:330; Duffy 1997; Trifiletti 1999) – although for different historical and cultural reasons.

7
Conclusions: Figuring Out the State of Professionalisation within European Health Care

This book has provided a broad comparative study of the implications of public management reforms for hospital doctors and nurses working within the public sector across Europe. It has concentrated on the interplay between certain of the core actors within the organisational network of hospital health care (doctors, nurses and patients) rather than a broader public administration or health policy approach. The underlying analysis has drawn on new institutionalism as a framework to facilitate comparative analysis although my approach has been somewhat ambivalent, reflecting a preference to view new institutionalism as a 'broad church', and from its doctrines I have drawn explicitly and implicitly the concepts of 'de-coupling', 'field' and 'sedimentation'[1] and have generally favoured the 'myth and ceremony' and social constructionist emphasis within the approach over more structuralist and a-historical elements as encapsulated in DiMaggio and Powell's (1991b) 'isomorphism' schema. For without being aware of the particular histories of medicine, nursing and the state, and of how their relations have variously negotiated, implicitly as well as explicitly, it is difficult to understand how particular organisational and managerial reforms might be responded to within particular societies. This point parallels Wilsford's notion of 'path dependency' (1994) and directly relates to the concept of 'governmentality', for the role of the medical profession as the dominant actor within the ensemble of health care expertise has been changing in varying degrees in different European countries, but particularly in France and the UK, in its interrelations with other professions, particularly nursing, and management. The general trend is towards sharpening the definition of autonomy, or 'loose-coupling', to apply more in the interests of managerial controls and less in terms of occupational autonomy.

There are two further points that emerge from these cross-European comparisons. First, is that the work and professional organisation of nurses is shaped more by state sponsorship than by any internally driven professionalisation project. Nursing as a professionalisation project is riven with fault lines as between 'carer' and 'practitioner' and it would appear that professionalisation for many nurses is a personal mission aimed at getting out of hospital work and into the community or the academy. Second, many patients too have a view on the provision of health care, and particularly those from a professional or white-collar background will for bad reasons as well as good will seek out private consultations in the view, apparently, that this will ensure a more convenient and better quality of care. The way in which each European country has planned or come to accept the configuration between the public and private delivery of health care has varied. The corporatist varieties of health services have incorporated private practice within their systems. The national health systems, whether of the quasi-liberal or Southern European varieties, have had more difficulty in finding a satisfactory solution to the challenge, and only the 'universalist' regimes of Scandinavia have in the past resolved the issue by ensuring the health care system is extremely well funded. With the universal recognition that public spending on health care has to be contained and cannot be left to rise inexorably year on year, all the European health care regimes have had to find ways of limiting the rise in this area. The challenge in part is how to do so constructively, that is, reconfiguring the division of labour and the sources and means of funding in ways that best suit the culture and social organisation of the various regimes. However, that has not been the brief of this book; rather my concern has been to describe and analyse the professional organisation of hospital-based medicine and nursing and their interrelations within the wider network of health care.

There are three further sections to this concluding chapter that reflect and extend the discussion so far: first, a discussion of the role of the patient within the actor-network of health care delivery; second, an overview of nursing across European identifying and restating key themes drawn from the case studies; third, a revisiting of the discussion on professional autonomy, dominance, loose-coupling and the health care state in light of the case studies to construct an alternative schema to begin to provide a means of comparing European health care organisations and professions and which recognises and begins to account for the historical, cultural, social as well as political dimensions to the processes of health care reforms across Europe.

Patients, nurses and doctors in Europe

The proto-professionalisation of patients

The reforms associated with new public management within health care have been aimed at bringing the cost and quality of health care more effectively under the control of the state. This has involved redefining the compact or contract between medicine, public and the state. Increasingly, accountability and quality are no longer an issue left to the organised profession to manage, and professional education and training are no longer deemed sufficient to inculcate good practice. Doctors in many European countries are now required to be re-accredited at regular intervals, to be seen to work in line with evidence-based practice and to have their work routinely evaluated according to criteria not necessarily of their own choosing. In this project the European states are claiming to give greater emphasis to the wishes of patients as users or consumers in pressing for improvements in care. One of the perverse problems for the reformers, given the claim that the patient is the core concern, has been the particularity of peoples' attachments towards their physical health and the apparent preference of sizeable segments of them across Europe to access specific doctors with known reputations, or at least doctors they believe have good reputations. De Swaan (1988:244–6) in his comparative study of Germany, Britain, France, US and Netherlands argues that patients have become 'proto-professionals'. This is achieved by means of a 'hidden curriculum' imbued at the clinic and consulting room and leading to 'a simplified and censored version of professional knowledge' (ibid.:244) which reflects the continuing 'medicalisation' of everyday life and drives people to seek reassurance as to the quality of the medical and health services available: 'professions do not simply force themselves upon innocent and unknowing clients...such persons or families usually have long since learned to define what bothers them in terms of some available proto-professional vocabulary' (de Swaan 1988:246).

If it is the case that patients and their families have concerns about the quality of the professional expertise available locally at least some of them will seek out what they believe to be the best, or the best they can afford. This could be within the private sector – as, for instance, in France or Britain – or within the 'subterranean economy' funded by 'little envelopes' as in Poland and Greece. In all these countries the practice, legitimate or illicit, is clientelistic in that the patient seeks the reassurance of obligation from their professional adviser as how to receive the best treatment. Where the publicly available services are particularly poor or limited the illicit payment of 'little envelopes' has less to do with buying medical obligation to the patient than in rationing medical care to those that can afford to pay for it. Both approaches enhance doctors' incomes. This proto-professionalism of patients and their families is profoundly medically focused and perhaps unaware of the potential contribution of nursing to health care services and even less to any health promotion campaigns. With proto-professionalism, the doctor always knows best, once you have found the right one.

European nursing professions

Nursing work, particularly within acute hospitals, rarely enjoys the autonomy and discretion often assumed to be the case with medical work. It is true that nursing remains much influenced by its oral tradition, which has only been partially superseded by the nursing theories that emanated out of North America from about the 1970s onwards (for example, George 1995). The degree to which these theories, especially relating to the 'nursing process',[2] have taken hold in the professional discourse within different European countries is related primarily to three interrelated factors: (1) emergence of academic 'professionalisers' within nursing (Melia 1987); (2) medical dominance; (3) and regime type (the state). To start with the last factor first, it is within the Breadwinner (corporatist) regimes (see Chapter 2) that nursing has distinct problems in establishing a professional base comparable to the Anglo-Saxon (liberal) regimes. This is because of the gendered consequences of having established the medical profession as the corporate and autonomous body legally responsible for the delivery of medical care. Even here, however, public management reforms have created organisational spaces for nurse managers within the hospitals. More generally, and across all regime types, the professional status, autonomy and influence of nursing is more dependent on the state than it is subject to medical dominance.

The influence of medical dominance on the work of nurses is in part rooted in the embedded values that gave rise, historically, to nursing as a distinct occupation. Nursing was defined as much on its role as medical helper as it was on patient care – an ambivalent ambiguity – which, as pointed out in Chapter 2, has tended to reflect a stratification of nursing into a not always well-integrated configuration of rank and file, clinical, academic and managerial elements with varying degrees of commitment to establish an autonomous professional jurisdiction for nursing. Within the Breadwinner (corporate) as well as Universalist (social democratic) regimes this autonomy has rested on claims of the separateness of patient care from treatment. In France this has become officially recognised, with nursing work being formally defined as comprising two elements, medically directed work and autonomous patient care work (see Chapter 4). Southern European nursing is in some ways similar to the Breadwinner model except, with a less well-organised medical profession, both state regulation and family expectations (familialism) play a larger role in defining the jurisdiction of nursing. For these reasons the formal professional organisation may be more developed, as is the case in Italy, than in the Breadwinner states (see Chapter 5). At the same time, the nurses' work situation within the Southern European countries remains very much more constrained than their colleagues in Germany, and other Breadwinner states. The case of nursing within the transitional states of Eastern Europe is similar in some respects to Southern Europe but, drawing here on Poland as the example (Chapter 6), it would appear that the trajectory may well be a different one with the direction of development more in line with the Breadwinner (corporate) states.

The Universalist regimes of Scandinavia might reasonably be considered the most likely location for an autonomous nursing profession, with its history and reputation for specialist nursing. But on a more detailed examination (Chapter 3) it turns out that the close interrelation between state and medicine has closed or limited the space for nurse autonomy. Even so, it would certainly appear to be the case that nurses' specialisation is experienced more as collaborative clinical working than simply the outcome of the medical domination of clinical work. It is the putative 'liberal' regime of the UK that has in many ways presented nurses with the greatest prospects of formal professionalisation and work autonomy, and it has been a state-driven agenda that has largely driven this project. Expanded nursing roles, nurse specialists and consultants have been more actively pursued by the UK state than by the organised profession. At the same time, nursing here is probably less dominated by medicine than in other European countries and the profession is less concerned than many of their colleagues within the corporate (Breadwinner) regimes to limit their claims for autonomy to nursing care only. It is probable that many nurses within the corporate regimes and in Southern Europe too do not view the hospital setting as the most favourable one for the development of professional nursing. Instead, they consider nursing within the community, possibly even more so than their Northern European colleagues, as the nursing domain within which they can most effectively develop professionally and practice autonomously. This issue has not been explored systematically here and would require further research to be able to assert with certainty.

The emergence of the academic professionaliser within nursing, in some important respects, cross-cuts the regime and medical dominance distinctions. In Northern Europe the nurse academic is broadly part of the professionalisation project of nurses and while relations between nursing 'segments' are hardly ever harmonious, there is a real sense that nursing departments within universities are working on the same broad project as those in clinical nursing. This would seem to be less the case in some of the corporate and particularly the Southern European regimes where, first, the universities are much more powerful 'actors' within the professional network and one that holds divergent interests to that of the practicing professionals. This is why the Italian nursing *collegi*, while welcoming their elevation to full professional standing as an *ordine*, resisted the relocation of nursing courses within the traditional universities (see Chapter 5). Second, the academic department can be seen as a means of attaining individual professional status and autonomy and as providing an escape route from restrictions of hospital nursing. This strategy was most apparent within Greece where hospital nursing enjoys low public esteem but can provide a career path to academic life with its associated higher public standing. Overall, however, the distinctions between the various regimes and nurse professionalisation must not be exaggerated, for while the differences are real they are more matters of degree than of kind. Equally, however, these differences do persist even when subjected to the isomorphic influences (coercive and normative) of European Commission regulations on nursing education and training and mobility of labour. But I would suggest that these are variations on a common set of themes captured by the notion of segmentation.

Medical dominance, the state and 'loosely-coupled' autonomy

The four case study chapters identified the variations in the organisation of the medical and nursing professions in the different countries and, in addition to presenting a description of acute hospital services within European health care systems, focused on specific themes particularly relevant to each of the case study comparisons. To reiterate from the introduction, these were as follows: accountability and clinical guidelines; state – professions relations and governmentality; federalism, regionalism and subsidiarity; clientelism and familialism. From this overarching review of themes it was possible to derive a model introduced initially in Chapter 6 that provided a map of medical dominance, managerial control and professional autonomy (see Figure 7.1).

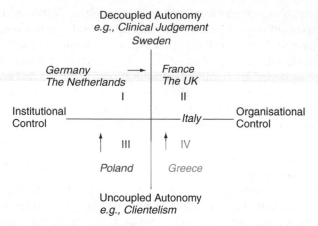

Figure 7.1   Loose coupling, professionalism and managerial control

Accounts of the changing status and autonomy of the medical profession have generally been around arguments of de-skilling, de-professionalisation and proletarianisation (see Chapter 2). In their different ways they have all pointed to the possibility that hospital doctors have become increasingly subject to external managerial control. What is clear from these case studies is that the medical profession enjoys a socially embedded status largely separate from issues of governmentality but links directly with the patient and their families and largely independent of state mediation. Meyer and Rowan's (1991) concept of decoupling is useful for accounting for the legitimated linkage between formal rules and professional practice. In fact, the discourse on the quality control of medical care, with its emphasis having shifted from professional self-regulation to managerial scrutiny, has clearly reconfigured the rules of decoupling. The Netherlands have relied on the rhetoric of clinical guidelines that were consensual within the profession, for example, while in the UK the preference has been for evidence-based medicine. In both cases it is clear that while the medical profession has to be more transparent in its approach to quality of care, nevertheless decoupling is essential to the effectiveness of the system. Simply put, there is not always 'one best way' for dealing with a medical problem, nor is there always good scientific evidence, yet the profession has to respond to a greater or lesser extent as if there were. There is another side to this 'loose-coupling' (Weick 1976), to use the more general term, whereby doctors will overcharge or charge illicit co-payments ('little brown envelopes', *fakelakia*), which is corrupting of the profession's contract with the state and compact with the patient. It is useful to put the two dimensions (control and loose-coupling) together to make up a two-by two-set of logically alternative cells (see Figure 7.1). This provides a means of contrasting professional versus state/managerial control on one axis, and type and degree of loose-coupling along the other. The horizontal axis discriminates between organisational versus institutional control (that is, managerial versus professional control) over medicine. The vertical axis distinguishes between 'decoupled autonomy' (legitimated autonomy, such as clinical judgement) and the illicit variety labelled here as 'uncoupled autonomy' (for example, accepting illicit co-payments). These axes represent continua and not discrete alternatives: institutional control may well co-exist in a symbiotic relation with organisational control (for example, Sweden). This is unlikely to be the case with uncoupled and decoupled autonomies, although an example would be where hospital doctors find the means to provide and prescribe a drug necessary for the care of a patient but not officially available (for example, see Chapter 6 re Poland). More generally, however, the illicit nature of uncoupled autonomy individuates the profession and rather than providing the substructure to collective professional autonomy either operates in its absence or undermines it. This figure is a representation and not an explanation but it does help map out the territory and provides a basis for comparison between European countries. The positioning of the six case study countries on Figure 7.1 is intended to represent their relative positions to each other but not with any precise mathematical accuracy. Thus Germany's and The Netherlands' hospital doctors occupy cell I representing the two countries where the profession enjoys the greatest institutionalised autonomy. France and the UK are placed in cell II because they both have been far more effectively subjected to state-led managerial reforms than any other European countries. Poland is located in cell III because, as in Germany, the medical profession has now its own 'chamber' as well as well-established infrastructure of scientific associations and has a long history of advising government on medical policy. At the same time, the practice of expecting illicit co-payments under the desk still exists and despite recent reforms may take time to eradicate from the system. Greece is in cell IV because the state-run health system accepts and relies on doctors accepting illicit co-payments (*fakelakia*) and working privately (even when this is technically illegal). Greece is one of the Southern European countries which shares certain cultural values and expectations with, at least, Southern Italy where there has also been a blurring of public and private provision of medical consultations. It is less clear how far these practices impacted on Northern Italy although the deeply rooted historical, social, political and economic differences would indicate that they are less affected. However, *partitocrazia* (Krause 1996), or political clientelism, has had a wide and systemic effect in undermining professional identity generally across Italy and for these reasons the country is located on the dividing line between cells II and IV. The case of medicine is here similar to nursing in as much as professional status is likely to be associated with an academic post within a university rather than as a practitioner. Finally, the Swedish profession is located straddling cells I and II to indicate its medical profession's long history of sustaining its status and autonomy by working directly from within the state apparatus.

The arrows marked on the diagram indicate the direction current policies are pushing the profession. Whether they are successful or not will depend in part on whether the other actors in the actor network also want this to happen and whether the states can find the means of funding the health systems sufficiently to meet the aspirations of all the players, which in health care is virtually an ontological impossibility.

Final comments

It is clear that European health systems have all been subjected to strong pressures for change. Initially, in the time-frame of this analysis, the incentive was to contain costs and, as exemplified by Sweden, to do so with the least political damage. The initial front-runner innovation was the regulated market with The Netherlands, the UK and Sweden leading the way. Each in their different ways adapted and modified the original 'marketisation' agenda until the simulacrum of a competitive marketplace gave way to variations on a managed care model. Enthoven's model was more about managed care based on HMOs than marketisation (Ranade 1998:7). At this time Germany was able to hold aloof and to do so for a long time, preferring to adapt its corporatist model to ensure tighter cost containment. These adaptations have provided alternative models for other European countries which share some of the cultural and social embeddedness of Germany, including Poland and Italy as well as The Netherlands in their retreat from the market.

The argument that has been presented here has been that the forces for convergence in European health care services have been seriously challenged by those deeply embedded social and cultural, as well as political, forces that have resisted, adapted and undermined attempts at managerial reforms. It is within this matrix of forces that the medical and nursing professions have been to varying degrees variously reshaped to better fit a health service characterised more by managed care than professional dominance.

Notes

1 Reorganising Hospital Medicine and Nursing in Europe

1 McGregor also goes on to argue for a radical alternative to the 'third way', although one that has several aims in common including 'decentralisation, local variation...joined up solutions...better informed governance' (1999:107). But this is shifting from analysis to prescription, which is not my concern at present.

2 All the case study countries were visited between 1996 and 2000 and a minimum of two hospitals was visited with a range of hospital doctors being interviewed in each, plus representatives of hospital management and senior nurse and/or nurses. Depending on local arrangements, national leaders, civil servants and academics were also interviewed (for example, Italy and Poland).

2 European Hospitals, Medicine, Nursing and Management

1 O'Connor (1996:22) cites Dalley (1988) in arguing that the hegemony of familialism not only is based on assumptions of the traditional (patriarchal) family but also reflects the philosophical tradition of 'possessive individualism' (Macpherson 1962) within which the individual is implicitly male.

2 Work situation is a Weberian concept used by Lockwood (1958) in his study of clerical workers. It refers to the social relations of the workplace and in that sense is similar to Braverman's (1974) Marxist concept of the 'labour process' (Abercrombie and Urry 1983:110).

3 The path dependency approach is discussed further in Chapter 3 in relation to French reforms of their health system.

3 The Netherlands and Sweden: Quality Control

1 Bartlett and Le Grand (1993) introduced the term 'quasi-market' on the grounds that it was more accurate than the term 'internal market', for these markets within health care were highly regulated and not concerned principally with profits but in improvements in efficiency.

2 Health Maintenance Organisations (HMO) are well established in the USA and are designed to provide 'managed care', that is, 'health care in as cost efficient a manner as possible, and the responsibility for attaining efficiency is shared by intermediaries that provide insurance or financing, physicians and [hospitals]' (Scott, Ruef, Mendel and Caronna 2000:41).

3 I am indebted to Jane Salvage (editor of *Nursing Times*) for providing me with a copy. The document is no longer available from the WHO (Regional Office for Europe) website.

4 For details of the developments in the Swedish health systems during the intervening years of the nineteenth and twentieth centuries see Immergut 1992:189–205.

5 It appears that *Primärvården* is the more commonly used term for what in the UK is referred to as the outpatients department (Berg, E. 2002). I will persist in using the term *polikliniks* as it is a term common across Europe (with slight differences in spelling).

6 The internal divisions within the Swedish medical profession were similar to those the French doctors faced with the not dissimilar *Débre* reforms of a decade earlier (see Chapter 4).

7 One consequence of the cost-containment policy was the re-emergence of a private health sector. While representing less than 2 per cent of acute beds in 1990 there were early indications that it was growing (Garpenby 1992:20) and has continued to do so. Diderichsen (1999:1157) reports that 20 per cent of hospital beds are now privately funded.

8 There are 21 county councils and three municipalities which make up the Federation of County Councils (*Landstingsförbundet*), an employee's organisation established in 1920s with a responsibility for health care provision and negotiating with the health unions (Garpenby 1999:409; European Observatory on Health Care Systems – Sweden 2001:15).

9 In a formal sense the specialty associations are also linked to the SMA. This is mainly for historical reasons – these associations are not part of the democratic structures of the SMA.

10 The Swedish Association of Hospital Physicians was previously known as *Overläkarföreningen.*

11 There are other authorities with responsibility in the health care sector, for example the Swedish Council on Technology Assessment in Health Care (SBU) which is responsible for strengthening the contribution of evidence-based health care, the Medical Products Agency and the national Social Insurance Board. The latter, however, now plays a smaller role than previously as the county councils become ever-increasingly responsible for the financing of health care in the public sector.

12 According to the *Nursing and Midwifery Profile: The Netherlands* (WHO 1996) there are 55 nurse organisations in total.

13 European directive 77/453/EEG.

14 I do not have any figures on the proportion of Dutch doctors who are female but the figure for the EC as a whole was around 26 per cent in the early 1990s and 50 per cent of those graduating from medical schools. It is estimated that in 2000 around one-third of all doctors were female (Brearley 1992:46).

4 United Kingdom and France: *Étatiste* Traditions

1 This discussion will complement that on The Netherlands and Sweden in the previous chapter. These four countries have been the most actively committed to the utilisation of clinical and health care guidelines out of the eight countries discussed in this book.

2 There were also 33,190 GPs plus 11,700 practice nurses (attached to GP practices) (European Observatory – UK 1999:81).

3 There is not a European Observatory on Health Care Systems for France.
4 The term 'organised profession' is used to denote an occupation whose practitioners are also necessarily members of a professional association and have to be registered in order to practice.
5 The per diem system was the common system by which hospitals were paid by the sickness funds across the corporatist regimes. An amount was agreed between the hospitals and sickness fund as a reasonable figure for each day a patient was in hospital. The problem with this model is that it provides a built in disincentive for the hospital to discharge patients early.

5 Germany and Italy: Federalism and Regionalism

1 There have been periodic attempts to change the status of these hospital associations and put them on an equal footing with the physicians associations but not with any success as yet (Busse *et al.* 1997).
2 Following the reunification of Germany there was an expectation in some quarters that ambulatory care would be provided by the hospitals as the East German health system relied on policlinic provision rather than independent (private) practitioners. By 1991, however, 'more than 80 per cent of outpatient doctors [based in Eastern Germany] had become office-based' and by 1993 'less than 5 per cent of outpatient doctors worked in polyclinics' (Wasem 1997:169).
3 *Krankenhausfinazierungsgesetz* (1972)
4 Interview carried out in German and translated by C. Preuschoft, November 2000, for a revised version of a paper (Dent *et al.* 2001) originally presented at the European Group for Organizational Studies (EGOS).
5 Translation provided by Claudia Preuschoft.
6 See Note 4.
7 The number has fallen slightly since then as a result of Lombardy further reducing its local health units by two-thirds to 15 (European Observatory – Italy: 2001:14)
8 The issues of clientelism and familialism are discussed in more detail in Chapter 6 on Greece and Poland. Only one aspect of clientelism will be discussed here in any detail and that is in connection with *partitocrazia*.
9 Fattore (1999) actually identifies four themes, the last being the right to opt out of the SSN. Initially individuals had the right to opt out provided they had sufficient private health insurance. These individuals would still have to pay their tax and other compulsory contributions but would receive a voucher to spend within the private sector. It was removed from the legislation in 1993.
10 One outcome of the reforms has been the rapid growth of the private health sector. It has been estimated that it may be meeting more than 30 per cent of the country's health needs (Fattore 1999:540). It is important to be reminded, however, that – similar to Germany – the private hospital sector is not dominated by for-profit institutions but by not-for-profit hospitals run by the Catholic Church.
11 There is some debate about the accuracy of DRGs as the system is based on studies of only eight hospitals mainly located in the North (Fattore 1999:536).

12 The establishment of an *ordine* for physicians in Italy was in advance of Germany where, despite pressures, the professional status of physicians was not fully resolved until 1935 (with the establishment of the national phys- icians' code) although *Ärtzekammern* were established in several *Land* before then (Moran 1999:38).

13 I was informed by a doctors' union (*sindacale*) leader in the Spring 2000 that a *numerus clausus* had now been introduced but was not expected to be strin- gently applied as this would undermine the position of the universities.

14 As in Italy there are nursing associations with religious affiliations – Catholic and Protestant.

15 These details were provided by the National Secretary of the *Federazione dei Collegi* and the President of Rome *Collegi* in March 2000.

16 The private sector is predominantly made up of Catholic hospitals and clinics located mainly in the south.

17 See Note 15.

18 Source same as fn. 17.

19 This interpretation is the one given by members of the nursing federation interviewed in March 2000.

20 This nurse works in a not-for-profit hospital with religious affiliation. While nursing work and organisation in both public and private hospitals are very similar it is possible that this tendency for nurses formally to carry out medical tasks is greater in the church hospitals. The rationale for this would be that public sector hospitals employ more doctors.

21 *Mansionerio*, from *mansione*, meaning 'task' or 'duty' (*Oxford Italian Dictionary*).

6 Poland and Greece: Transition or Embeddedness?

1 The political programme for Greek nationalism came importantly from the Greek *diaspora* (Mouzelis 1986:41), especially the traders who settled in Continental Europe. This merchant class were responsible for importing the ideals of the French Revolution that underpinned the struggle for independence, a struggle in which the British, French and Russians played a significant role in imposing 'change from above' (Katrougalos 1996:44).

2 The sickness funds also provide sickness benefits and most maternity benefits, spa treatment and funeral expenses too, although provision varies greatly between the funds.

3 The pre-existing system of health care was based on social insurance (sickness funds) – corporatist – model (Liaropoulos and Kaitelidou 1997:3).

4 This information was provided by a member of the group in a telephone interview that took place in May 1998.

5 The Centre of Health System Management research is part of a broader programme of raising awareness of consumer rights and includes what was referred to as 'institutional bribes' for donations to foundations as well as those from private individuals. Moreover, data of this kind needs to be interpreted very carefully as respondents may not wish to confess to making 'illegal' payment or conversely, for political purposes, overstate any such payments.

6 According to a newspaper report in December 1998 (TA NEA 1998:16) the average physician – population ratio is 1:201. Within Greece the physician – population ratios reflect great inequality as between Athens, at 1:170, and the rest of Greece. The ratio for Central Macedonia and Thessolonika is 1:236, and for Western Greece 1:349. These figures contrast markedly with the 1:567 in the Peloponnese and 1:630 in Central Greece (see also WHO – Greece 1996:48). Athens is the honeypot of Greek medicine: 54 per cent of all physicians work in the conurbation while only 3 per cent are employed in Central Greece. (Dr Samatas, University of Crete, kindly provided the English translation of this and the other Greek-language newspapers referred to in this chapter.)

7 'Habilitation' is the qualification for professor status in countries organised similarly to Germany. It is, apparently, a little like presenting a second thesis.

7 Conclusions: Figuring Out the State of Professionalisation within European Health Care

1 These concepts are explained in Chapter 2.
2 The 'nursing process' model is described in Chapter 5 (Italy and Germany).

Bibliography

Abbott, A. (1988) *The System of Professions: An Essay on the Division of Expert Labour*. Chicago and London: The University of Chicago Press.

Abbott, P. and Giarchi, G. G. (1997) 'Health, Healthcare and Health Inequalities', in T. Spybey (ed.) *Britain in Europe: An Introduction to Sociology*, London: Routledge, 359–78.

Abel-Smith, B., Calltorp, J., Dixon, M., Dunning, A., Evans, R., Holland, W. W., Jarman, B. and Mossialos, E. (1994) *Report on Greek Health Services*, Athens: Ministry of Health and Social Welfare of Greece, Pharmétrica SA.

Abercrombie, N. and Urry, J. (1983) *Capital, Labour and the Middle Classes*, London: George Allen & Unwin.

Altenstetter, C. (1989) 'Hospital Planners and Medical Professionals in the Federal Republic of Germany', in G. Freddi and J. W. Björkman (eds), *Controlling Medical Professionals: The Comparative Politics of Health Governance*, London: Sage, 157–77.

Altenstetter, C. (1997) 'Health Policy Making in Germany', in C. Altenstetter and J. W. Björkman (eds) *Health Policy Reform, National Variations and Globalization*, Basingstoke: Macmillan, 136–60.

Altenstetter, C. and Björkman, J. W. (eds) (1997) *Health Policy Reform, National Variations and Globalization*, Basingstoke: Macmillan – now Palgrave Macmillan.

Armongathe, J. F. (1989) *Towards the Development of Medical Evaluation: Report to the Ministry of Solidarity, Health and Social Welfare*, Paris: La Documentation Française.

Athens News (1999) 'Simitis Stresses Unity, Vows to Win Euro Polls: Combative PM Peppers Speech with Populist Rhetoric', 19 March, 3.

Axelsson, R. (2000) 'The Organizational Pendulum: Healthcare Management in Sweden 1865–1998', *Scandinavian Journal of Public Health*, 28, 47–53.

Bagguley, P. (1994) 'Prisoners of the Beveridge Dream? The Political Mobilisation of the Poor Against Contemporary Welfare Regimes', in R. Burrows and B. Loader (eds) *Towards a Post-Fordist Welfare State?* London: Routledge, 74–94.

Barley, S. R. (1986) 'Technology as an Occasion for Structuring: Evidence from Observations of CT Scanners and the Social Order of Radiology Departments', *Administrative Science Quarterly* 31, 78–108.

Barley, S. R. and Tolbert, P. S. (1997) 'Institutionalisation and Structuration: Studying the Links between Action and Institution', *Organization Studies* 18/1, 93–117.

Bartlett, W. and Le Grand, J. (1993) 'The Theory of Quasi-Markets', in J. and Le Grand and W. Bartlett (eds) *Quasi-Markets and Social Policy*, London: Macmillan 13–34.

Benner, P. (1984) *From Novice to Expert: Excellence and Power in Clinical Nursing Practice*, London: Addison-Wesley.

Bentling, S. (1992) *I idéernas värld: en analys av omvårdnad som vetenskap och grund för en professionell utbildning (Uppsala)* [An Analysis of Nursing and Caring as a Basis for Professional Training], Uppsala: Uppsala Studies in Education 45.

Berg, E. (2002) *Personal communication*, 12 November, Luleå University of Technology, Sweden.

Berg, M. (2001) *Personal Communication*, 30 September, BMG, Erasmus University, Rotterdam, The Netherlands.

Berg, M. and van der Grinten, T. (forthcoming) 'Priority Setting in Dutch Health Care', in C. Ham (ed.) *Priority Setting in Health Care*, Buckingham: Open University Press.

Berger, P. L. and Luckman, T. (1967) *The Social Construction of Reality*, Harmondsworth: Penguin.

Berlant, J. L. (1975) *Profession and Monopoly: A Study of Medicine in the United States and Great Britain*, Los Angeles and London: University of California Press.

Björkman, J. W. and Okma, K. G. H. (1997) 'Restructuring the Health Care Systems in The Netherlands: The Institutional Heritage of Dutch Health Policy Reforms', in C. Altenstetter and J. W. Björkman (eds) *Health Policy Reform, National Variations and Globalization*, Basingstoke: Macmillan Press – now Palgrave, 79–108.

Bouget, D. (1998) 'The Juppé Plan and the Future of the French Social Welfare System', *Journal of European Social Policy*, 8(2), 155–72.

Bourdieu, P. (1977) *Outline of a Theory of Practice*, Cambridge: Cambridge University Press.

Braverman, H. (1974) *Labor and Monopoly Capitalism: The Degradation of Work in the Twentieth Century*, New York: Monthly Review Press.

Brunni, A. and Gheradi, S. (2002) 'Omega's Story: The Heterogeneous Engineering of a Gendered Professional Self', in M. Dent and S. Whitehead (eds) *Managing Professional Identities: Knowledge, Performativity and the 'New' Professional*, London: Routledge, 174–98.

Brykczynska, G. (1992) 'Nurse Education in Poland', *Senior Nurse*, 12(1), 21–4.

Bucher, R. and Strauss, A. (1961) 'Professions in Process', *American Journal of Sociology*, 66, 325–34.

Burrage, M., Jaurausch, K. and Siegrist, H. (1990) 'An Actor-based Framework for the Study of the Profession', in M. Burrage and R. Torstendahl (eds) *Professions in Theory and History*, London: Sage, 203–25.

Busse, R. and Howorth, C. (1999) 'Cost Containment in Germany: Twenty Years Experience', in E. Mossialos and J. Le Grand (eds) *Health Care and Cost Containment in the European Union*, Aldershot: Ashgate: 303–39.

Busse, R. Howorth, C. and Schwartz, F. W. (1997) 'The Future Development of the Rights Based Approach to Health Care in Germany: More Rights or Fewer?', in Lenaghan, J. (ed.) *Hard Choices in Health Care* London: BMJ Publishing.

Butler, J. (1990) *Gender Trouble: Feminism and the Subversion of Identity*, London: Routledge.

Butler, J. (2002) *Personal communication*, Department of Public Health (*Abteilung Gesudheit und Soziales*), Berlin.

Cabinet Office/Department of Health (2002) *'Making a Difference': Reducing Burdens in Hospital*, London: Public Sector Team, available at www.cabinetoffice.gov.uk/regulation/publicsector/index.htm.

Callon, M. (1986) 'Some Elements of a Sociology of Translation: Domestication of the Scallops and the Fishermen of St Brieuc Bay', in J. Law (ed.) *Power, Action and Belief: a New Sociology of Knowledge?* London: Routledge and Kegan Paul, 196–233.

Carpenter, M. (1977) 'The New Managerialism and Professionalism in Nursing', in M. Stacey, M. Reid and R. Dingwall (eds) *Health and the Division of Labour*, London: Croom Helm, 165–95.

Cartwright, F. F. (1977) *A Social History of Medicine*, London: Longman.

Casparie, A. F. (1991) 'Guidelines to Shape Clinical Practice: The Role of Medical Societies – the Dutch Experience in Comparison with Recent Developments in the American Approach', *Health Policy*, 18, 251–9.

Casparie, A. F. (1993) 'View from The Netherlands', *Quality in Health Care*, 2, 138–41.

Casparie, A. F. (1995) 'Medical Audit in The Netherlands: Experience Over 22 Years', *Journal of Epidemiology and Community Health*, 49, 557–8.

Chawla, M., Berman, P. and Kawiorska, D. (1998) 'Financing Health Services in Poland: New Evidence on Private Expenditures', *Health Economics*, 7, 337–46.

Clarke, J. and Newman, J. (1997) *The Managerial State*, London: Sage.

Clegg, S. (1989) *Frameworks of Power*, London: Sage.

Cochrane, A. L. (1972) *Effectiveness and Efficiency: Random Reflections on Health Services*, London: Nuffield Provincial Hospital Trust.

Colombotos, J. and Fakiolas, N. P. (1993) 'The Power of Organized Medicine in Greece', in F. W. Hafferty and J. B. McKinlay (eds) *The Changing Medical Profession: an International Perspective*, New York and Oxford: Oxford University Press, 138–231.

Cooper, D. J., Hinings, C. R., Greenwood, R. and Brown, J. L. (1996) 'Sedimentation and Transformation in Organizational Change: The Case of Canadian Law Firms', *Organizational Studies*, 17(4), 623–47.

Cox, D. (1991) 'Health Service Management – a Sociological View: Griffiths and the Non-Negotiated Order of the Hospital', in J. Gabe, M. Calnan and M. Bury (eds) *The Sociology of the Health Service*, London: Routledge, 89–114.

Czapinski, J. and Panek, T. (2000) *Social Diagnosis*, Warsaw: Department of the Prime Minister.

Dalley, G. (1988) *Ideologies of Caring: Rethinking Community and Collectivism*, London: Macmillan Press – now Palgrave,.

Davies, C. (1995) *Gender and the Professional Predicament in Nursing*, Buckingham: Open University Press.

Davies, C. (1996) 'The Sociology of the Professions and the Profession of Gender', *Sociology*, 30(4), 661–78.

Davies, C. (2000) 'Getting Health Professionals to Work Together', *British Medical Journal (BMJ)*, 320, 1021–2.

Dechanoz, G. (1990) 'Challenges to Practice in France', in C. M. Fagin (ed.) *Nursing Leadership*, National League for Nursing Publications, 41 (2349), 155–61.

Dekker, W. (1987) *Willingness to Change*, The Hague: SDU.

de Kervasdoué, J., Meyer, C., Weill, C. and Couffinahl, A. (1997) 'The French Health Care System: Inconsistent Regulation', in C. Altenstetter and S. W. Björkman (eds) *Health Policy Reform, National Variations and Globalization*, Basingstoke: Macmillan Press – now Palgrave, 59–78.

Dent, M. (1993) 'Professionalism, Educated Labour and the State: Hospital Medicine and the New Managerialism', *The Sociological Review*, 41(2), 244–73.

Dent, M. Howorth, H. Mueller, F. and Preuschoft, C. (2001) 'Archetype Transition in the German Health Service? The Attempted Modernisation of Hospitals in a North German State', paper presented at 17th EGOS, Lyon, 5–7 July.

Dent, M. and Whitehead, S. (2002) *Managing Professional Identities: Knowledge, Performativity and the 'New' Professional*, London: Routledge.

Department of Health (1989) *Working for Patients* (Cmnd 555), London: HMSO.

Department of Health (1994) *The Evolution of Clinical Audit* (Chair: M. Edwards, Regional Nurse Research and Development, Wessex Regional Health Authority), Heywood: The Health Publications Unit.

Department of Health (2000) *The New NHS – Modern, Dependable* (Cmmd 3807), London: The Stationary Office.

Department of Health (2001a) *Shifting the Balance of Power Within the NHS: Securing Delivery*, London: Department of Health, available at www.doh.gov.uk/shiftingthebalance

Department of Health (2001b) *Modernising Regulation in the Health Professions: Consultation Document*, London: Department of Health.

Department of Health (2002) *Modern Matrons in the NHS: A Progress Report*, London: Department of Health Publications, available at www.doh.gov.uk

de Pouvourville, G. (1997) 'Quality of Care Initiatives in the French Context', *International Journal for Quality in Health Care*, 9(3), 163–70.

de Pouvourville, G. (1998) *Personal communication*, March, Paris.

de Swaan, A. (1988) *In Care of the State*, Cambridge: Polity.

Derber, C. (1982) *Professionals as Workers: Mental Labor in Advanced Capitalism*, Boston, MA: G. K. Hall and Co.

Derber, C., Schwartz, W. A., Magrass, Y. (1990) *Power in the Highest Degree*, Oxford: Oxford University Press.

Dewar, S. and Finlayson, B. (2002) 'Regulating the Regulators', *BMJ*, 324, 378–9.

DGS/DHOS (2002a) *Nurse – Sommaire*, August available at www.sante.gouv.fr/htm

DGS/DHOS (2002b) *Infirmier Anesthésiste* [Nurse Anaesthetist] – *Sommaire*, August, available at www.sante.gouv.fr/htm

DGS/DHOS (2002c) *Infirmierde Bloc Opératoire* [Operating Theatre Nurse] – *Sommaire*, August, available at www.sante.gouv.fr/htm

DGS/DHOS (2002d) *Puéricultrice* [Paediatric Nurse] – *Sommaire*, August, available at www.sante.gouv.fr/htm

DGS/DHOS (2002e) *Directeur des Soins* [Director of the Care] – *Sommaire*, August, available at www.sante.gouv.fr/htm

Diderichsen, F. (1999) 'Devolution in Swedish Health Care', *BMJ*, 318, 1156–7.

DiMaggio, P. and Powell, W. W. (1991a) 'Introduction' in W. W. Powell and P. J. DiMaggio (eds) *The New Institutionalism in Organizational Analysis*, Chicago and London: The University of Chicago Press, 1–38.

DiMaggio, P. and Powell, W. W. (1991b) 'The Iron Cage Revisited: Institutional Isomorphism and Collective Rationality in Organizational Fields', in W. W. Powell and P. J. DiMaggio (eds) *The New Institutionalism in Organizational Analysis*, Chicago and London: The University of Chicago Press, 63–82.

Donozynski, A. (1998) 'France Moves Towards a GP System', *BMJ*, 317, 1545.

Dowie, R. and Langman, M. (1999) 'Staffing of Hospitals: Future Needs, Future Provision', *BMJ*, 319, 1193–5.

Duffy, D. M. (1997) 'State, Economy and Civil Society Interdependency', in C. Altenstetter and J. W. Björkman (eds) *National Policy Reform, National Variations and Globalization*, London: Macmillan Press – now Palgrave, 279–313.

Eckstein, H. (1958) *The English Health Service*, Cambridge, MA, Harvard University Press.

Eddy, D. M. (1990a) 'Guidelines for Policy Statements: the Explicit Approach', *Journal of the American Medical Association (JAMA)*, 263, 2239–443.

Eddy, D. M. (1990b) 'Designing a Practice Policy: Standards, Guidelines and Options, *JAMA*, 263, 3077–84.

ELEFTHEROTYPIA (*Freepress*) 'Third World Situation in 59 Major Greek Hospitals', 13 January, 16.

Ellwood, P. M. (1988) 'Outcomes Management; a Technology of Patient Experience', *New England Journal of Medicine*, 318, 1549–56

Elston, M. A. (1991) 'The Politics of Professional Power: Medicine in a Changing Health Service', in J. Gabe, M. Calnan and M. Bury (eds) *The Sociology of the Health Service*, London: Routledge, 58–88.

Enthoven, A. (1978) 'Consumer Choice Health Plan: A National Health Insurance Proposal Based on Regulated Competition in the Private Sector', *New England Journal of Medicine*, 298, (13), 709–20.

Enthoven, A. (1985) *Reflections on the Management of the National Health Service: An American Looks at Incentives to Efficiency in Health Services Management in the UK*, London: Nuffield Provincial Hospitals.

Enthoven, A. (1989) *Management Information Systems and Analysis of the Swedish Healthcare System*, Lund: IHE.

Esping-Andersen, G. (1990) *The Three Worlds of Welfare Capitalism*, Cambridge: Polity.

Esping-Andersen, G. (1996) 'After the Golden Age? Welfare State Dilemmas in a Global Economy', in G. Esping-Andersen (ed.) *Welfare States in Transition: National Adaptations in Global Economies*, London, Sage 1–31.

European Commission: Internal Market Directorate (Reference XV/98/09/E) (2000) *Study of Specialist Nurses in Europe*, Brussels, 1 August, MARKT/D/8031/2000.

European Observatory on Health Care Systems (1996) *Health Care Systems in Transition: Greece*, Copenhagen: WHO, Regional Office for Europe, available at www.euro.who.int/document/e72454.pdf

European Observatory on Health Care Systems (1999) *Health Care Systems in Transition: United Kingdom*, Copenhagen: WHO, Regional Office for Europe, available at www.euro.who.int/document/e68283.pdf

European Observatory on Health Care Systems (1999) *Health Care Systems in Transition: Poland*, Copenhagen: WHO, Regional Office for Europe, available at www.euro.who.int/document/e67136.pdf

European Observatory on Health Care Systems (2000) *Health Care Systems in Transition: Germany*, Copenhagen: WHO, Regional Office for Europe, available at www.euro.who.int/document/e68952.pdf

European Observatory on Health Care Systems (2001) *Health Care Systems in Transition: Sweden*, Copenhagen: WHO, Regional Office for Europe, available at www.euro.who.int/document/e73430.pdf

European Observatory on Health Care Systems (2001) *Health Systems in Transition: Italy*, Copenhagen: WHO, Regional Office for Europe, available at www.euro.who.int/document/e73096.pdf

Eurostat (1996) *Demographic Statistics*, Luxembourg: Office for Official Publications of the European Communities.

Exworthy, M. and Halford, S. (eds) (1999) *Professionals and the New Managerialism in the Public Sector*, Buckingham: Open University Press.

Fairfield, G., Hunter, D. J., Mechanic, D. and Rosleff, F. (1997) 'Managed Care: Origins, Principles, and Evolution', *BMJ*, 314, 1823, available at www.bmj.com

Fattore, G. (1999) 'Cost Containment and Reforms in the Italian NHS', in E. Mossialos and J. Le Grand (eds) *Cost Containment in the EU*, Aldershot: Ashgate, 513–46.

Ferrera, M. (1995) 'The Rise and Fall of Democratic Universalism: Health Care Reform in Italy, 1978–1994', *Journal of Health Politics, Policy and Law*, 20, 2, 275–302.

Ferrera, M. (1996) 'The Southern Model of Welfare in Social Europe', *Journal of European Social Policy*, 6, (1), 17–37.

Figueras, J., Saltman, R. B. and Sakellarides, C. (1998) 'Introduction', in R. B. Saltman, J. Figueras and C. Sakellarides (eds) *Critical Challenges for Health Care Reform in Europe*, Buckingham: Open University Press, 1–19.

Flynn, R. (1992) *Structures of Control in Health Management*, London: Routledge.

Foucault, M. (1973) *The Birth of the Clinic*, London: Tavistock.

Foucault, M. (1979a) *Discipline and Punish*, Harmondsworth: Penguin.

Foucault, M. (1979b) 'On Governmentality', *Ideology and Consciousness*, 6, 5–22.

Foucault, M. (1981) *History of Sexuality: an Introduction*, Harmondsworth: Penguin.

Foucault, M. (1991) 'Governmentality', in G. Burchill, C. Gordon and P. Miller (eds) *The Foucault Effect: Studies in Governmentality*, London: Harvester-Wheatsheaf, 87–104.

Fournier, V. (1999) 'The Appeal of "Professionalism" as a Disciplinary Mechanism', *The Sociological Review*, 47, (2), 280–307.

Fournier, V. (2000) 'Boundary Work and the (Un)making of the Profession', in Nigel Malin (ed.) *Professionalism, Boundaries and the Workplace*, London: Routledge, 67–86.

Freddi, G. (1989) 'Problems of Organisational Rationality in Health Systems: Political Controls and Policy Options', G. Freddi and J.W. Björkman (eds) *Controlling Medical Professionals: The Comparative Politics of Health Governance*, London: Sage, 1–27.

Freidson, E. (1994) *Professionalism Reborn: Theory, Prophecy and Policy*, Cambridge: Polity.

Friedman, A. L. (1977) *Industry and Labour*, London: Macmillan.

Garpenby, P. (1992) 'The Transformation of the Swedish Health Care System, or the Hasty Rejection of the Rational Planning Model', *Journal of European Social Policy*, 2, (1), 17–31.

Garpenby, P. (1999) 'Resource Dependency, Doctors and the State: Quality Control in Sweden', *Social Science & Medicine*, 49, 405–24.

Garpenby, P. (2002) *Personal Communication* (17 October 2002), Linköping University, Sweden.

Geertz, C. (1992) 'The Bazaar Economy: Information and Search in Peasant Marketing', in M. Granovetter and R. Swedberg (eds) *The Sociology of Economic Life*, Boulder, San Francisco and Oxford: Westview Press, 225–32.

George, J. B. (1995) *Nursing Theories: The Base for Professional Nursing Practice* (4th edn), London: Prentice-Hall International.

Giaimo, S. and Manow, P. (1997) 'Institutions and Ideas into Politics: Health Care Reform in Britain and Germany', in C. Altenstetter and J. W. Björkman (eds) *Health Policy Reform, National Variations and Globalization*, Basingstoke: Macmillan Press – now Palgrave, 175–202.

Giddens, A. (1984) *The Constitution of Society*, Cambridge: Polity.

Giddens, A. (1987) *Social Theory and Modern Sociology*, Cambridge: Polity.

Giddens, A. (1991) *The Consequences of Modernity*, Cambridge: Polity.

Godt, P. J. (1987) 'Confrontation, Consent, and Corporatism: State Strategies and the Medical Profession in France, Great Britain, and West Germany', *Journal of Health Politics, Policy and Law*, 12, (3), 459–80.

Goodin, R. E. and Rein, M. (2001) 'Regime on Pillars: Alternative Welfare State Logics and Dynamics', *Public Administration*, 79, (4), 769–801.

Gramsci, A. (1971) *Selections from the Prison Notebook*, edited and translated by Q. Hoare and G. N. Smith, London: Lawrence and Wishart, 5–23.

Granovetter, M. (1992) 'Economic Action and Social Structure: The Problem of Embeddedness', in M. Granovetter and R. Swedberg (eds) *The Sociology of Economic Life*, Boulder, San Francisco and Oxford: Westview Press, 53–81.

Greenwood, R. and Hinings, C. R. (1993) 'Understanding Strategic Change: The Contribution of Archetypes', *Academy of Management Journal*, 36, (5), 1052–81.

Griffiths, R. (1983) *National Health Service Management Inquiry*, 6 October London: Department of Health and Social Security.

Griggs, S. (1999) *Professionalisation, Policy Networks and the Development of French Health Policy: The Rise of Hospital Directors, The* Syndicat National des Cadres Hospitaliers, *1976–1991*, PhD thesis, Department of Government, London School of Economics and Political Science.

Griggs, S. and Dent, M. (1996) *Remodelling Public Hospitals in France and the UK*, (Knowledge, Organisations and Society Occasional Paper Series) Stoke on Trent: Staffordshire University.

Griggs, S. and Radcliffe, J. (1994) 'Bridging the Gap between Planning and Markets: Regulating Public Hospitals in UK and France', *Medical Law International*, 1, 231–44.

Guardian (1999) 'French Politicians on Trial for Mass AIDs Infection', Jon Henley, 6 February, 20.

Guardian (2000) 'Controversial Health List Ranks Britain 18th in World', 221 June: 3.

Guardian (2002) 'Main Points', 18 April, 17.

Habermas, J. (1976) 'Problems of Legitimation in Late Capitalism', in P. Connerton (ed) *Critical Sociology*, Harmondsworth: Penguin, 363–87.

Hajen, L., Paetow, P. and Schumacher, H. (2000) *Gesundheitsökonomie*, Stuttgart: 2000 Kapitel 7, Seite.

Ham, C. (ed.) (1997) *Health Care Reform: Learning from International Experience*, Buckingham: Open University Press.

Ham, C., Robinson, R. and Benzeval, M. (1990) *Health Check: Health Care Reforms in an International Context*, London: King's Fund Institute.

Hamburgische Krankenhausgessellschaft (1999) Hamburg: Krankenhausführer Hamburg.

Hanlon, G. (1998) 'Professionalism as Enterprise: Service Class Politics and the Redefinition of Professionalism', *Sociology*, 32, (1), 43–63.

Harrison, M. I. and Calltorp, J. (2000) 'The Reorientation of Market-Oriented Reforms in Swedish Health Care', *Health Policy*, 50, 219–40.

Harrison, M. I. and Lieverdink, H. (2000) 'Controlling Medical Specialists: Hospital Reforms in The Netherlands', *Research in the Sociology of Health Care*, 17, 63–79.

Harrison, S. (1999) 'Clinical Autonomy and Health Policy: Past and Futures', in M. Exworthy and S. Halford (eds) *Professionals and the New Managerialism in the Public Sector*, Buckingham: Open University Press, 50–64.

Harrison, S. and McDonald, R. (2003) 'Science, Consumerism and Bureaucracy: New Legitimations of Medical Professionalism', *International Journal of Public Sector Management* (forthcoming).

Havelková, H. (1993) '"Patriarchy" in Czech Society' *Hypatia*, 8, (4), 89–96.

Hearn, J. (1982) 'Notes on Patriarchy, Professionalization and the Semi-Professions', *Sociology*, 16, 184–201.

Herzlich, C. (1982) 'The Evolution of Relations Between French Physicians and the State from 1880 to 1980', *Sociology of Health and Illness*, 4, (3), 241–53.

Hood, C. (1991) 'A Public Management for All Seasons?' *Public Administration*, 69, 3–19.

Hood, C. (1995) 'The "New Public Management" in the 1980s: Variations on a Theme', *Accounting, Organizations and Society*, 20, 2, (3), 93–109.

Hood, C., Scott, C., James, O., Jones, G. and Travers, T. (1999) *Regulation Inside Government: Waste-Watchers, Quality-Police and Sleaze-Busters*, Oxford: Oxford University Press.

Horellou-Lefarge, C., Joncour, Y., and Lararge, H. (1990) 'Budget Global et Départmentalisations', *Gestions Hospitaliéres*, 294, 223–58.

Immergut, E. M. (1992) *Health Politics: Interests and Institutions in Western Europe*, Cambridge: Cambridge University Press.

Internal Document – *Vorstandssprecher* (1998) *Modernity Through FIT*, LBK, Management Letter, 2000, (1), 4–7.

Jacobs, A. (1998) 'Seeing Difference: Market Health Reform in Europe', *Journal of Health Politics, Policy and Law*, 23, (1), 1–33.

Jamous, H. and Peloille, B. (1970) 'Professions or Self-Perpetuating Systems? Changes in the French University-Hospital System', in J. A. Jackson (ed.) *Professions and Professionalization*, Cambridge: Cambridge University Press, 109–52.

Jary, D. (2002) 'Aspects of the "Audit Society": Issues arising from the Colonization of Professional Academic Identities by a "Portable Management Tool"', in M. Dent and S. Whitehead (eds) *Managing Professional Identities: Knowledge, Performativity and the 'New' Professional*, London: Routledge, 38–60.

Johnson, T. (1995) 'Governmentality and the Institutionalization of Expertise', in T. Johnson, G. Larkin and M. Saks (eds) *Health Professions and the State in Europe*, London: Routledge, 7–24.

Johnson, T. Larkin, G. and Saks, M. (eds) (1995) *Health Professions and the State in Europe*, London: Routledge.

Johnson, T. J. (1972) *Professions and Power*, London: Macmillan – now Palgrave.

Jost, T. S. (1990) *Assuring the Quality of Medical Practice: an International Comparative Study*, London: King Edward's Hospital Fund for London.

Jost, T. S. (1992) 'Recent Developments in Medical Quality Assurance and Audit: an International Comparative Study', in R. Dingwall and P. Fenn (eds) *Quality and Regulation in Health Care: International Experiences*, London: Routledge, 69–88.

Kanavos, P. and McKee, M. (1998) 'Macroeconomic Constraints and Health Challenges Facing European Health Systems', in R. B. Saltman, J. Figueras and C. Sakellarides (eds) *Critical Challenges for Health Care Reform in Europe*, Buckingham: Open University Press, 23–52.

Katrougalos, G. S. (1996) 'The South European Welfare Model: The Greek Welfare State, In Search of an Identity', *Journal of European Social Policy*, 6, (1), 39–60.

Katz, F. E. (1969) 'Nurses', in A. Etzioni (ed.) *The Semi-Professions and Their Organization: Teachers, Nurses, Social Workers*, New York: The Free Press, 54–81.

Kennedy, M. D. and Sadkowski, K. (1991) 'Constraints on Professional Power in Soviet-Type Society: Insights From the 1980–1981 'Solidarity' Period in Poland', in A. Jones (ed) *Professions and the State: Expertise and Autonomy in the Soviet Union and Eastern Europe*, Philadelphia: Temple University Press, 167–206.

Kennedy Report (2001) *The Report of the Public Inquiry into Children's Heart Surgery at the Bristol Royal Infirmary 1984–1995*, CM 5207[I] London: the Stationery Office, available at www.bristol-inquiry.org.uk/final report/index.htm

Kirkman-Liff, B. (1997) 'The United States', in C. Ham (ed.) *Health Care Reform: Learning from International Experience*, Buckingham: Open University Press, 21–45.

Kitchener, M. (1998) 'Quasi-Market Transformation: An Institutionalist Approach to Change in UK Hospitals', *Public Administration*, 76 (Spring), 73–95.

Klazinga, N. (1994) Compliance with Practice Guidelines: Clinical Autonomy Revisited', *Health Policy*, 28, 51–66.

Klazinga, N. (1996) *Quality Management of Medical Specialist Care in The Netherlands: an Explorative Study of its Nature and Development*, Den Haag: Belvédère.

Klein, R. (1995) 'Big Bang Health Reform – Does it Work?: The Case of UK's 1991 National Health Service Reforms, *The Milbank Quarterly*, 73, 299–338.

Klein, R. (2001) *The New Politics of the NHS* (4th edn), London: Prentice Hall.

Knox, R. A. (1993) *Germany: One Nation with Health Care for All*, Washington DC: Faulkner and Gray's Healthcare Information Center.

Kokko, S., Hava, P., Ortun, V. and Leppo, K. (1998) 'The Role of the State in Health Care Reform', in R. B. Saltman, J. Figueras and C. Sakellarides (eds) *Critical Challenges for Health Care Reform in Europe*, Buckingham: Open University Press, 289–307.

Kozierkiewicz, A. and Karski, J. B. (2001) 'Hospital Sector Reform in Poland', *Eurohealth*, 17, (3), 32–5.

Krause, E. A. (1996) *Death of the Guilds: Professions, States and the Advance of Capitalism, 1930 to the Present*, New Haven and London: Yale University Press.

Kutzin, J. (1998) 'The Appropriate Role for Patient Cost Sharing', in R. B. Saltman, J. Figueras and C. Sakellarides (eds) *Critical Challenges for Health Care Reform in Europe*. Buckingham: Open University Press, 78–112.

Kyriopoulas, J. E. and Tsalikis, G. (1993) 'Public and Private Imperatives of Greek Health Policies', *Health Policy*, 26, 105–117.

Lanara, V. (1996) 'Nursing Education in a United Europe: The Greek Case', *European Nurse*, 1, (1), 37–47.

Lancry, P-J. and Sandier, S. (1999) 'Twenty Years of Cures for the French Health Care System', in E. Mossialos and J. Le Grand (eds) *Health Care and Cost Containment in the European Union*, Aldershot: Ashgate, 443–71.

Landesbetrieb Krankenhauser (LBK) (1998) *Geschäftsbericht 1998* [Financial Report], Hamburg.

Lane, J-K, and Arvidson, S. (1989) 'Health Professionals in the Swedish System', in G. Freddi and J. W. Warner (eds) *Controlling Medical Professionals: the Comparative Politics of Health Governance*, London: Sage, 74–98.

Larkin, G. (1983) *Occupational Monopoly and Modern Medicine*, London: Tavistock.

Larkin, G. (1995) 'State Control and the Health Profession in the United Kingdom', in T. Johnson, G. Larkin and M. Saks (eds) *Health Professions and the State in Europe*, London: Routledge, 45–54.

Larson, M. S. (1977) *The Rise of Professionalism: A Sociological Analysis*, Berkeley, Los Angeles and London: University of California Press.

Larson, M. S. (1980) 'Proletarianisation and Educated Labor', *Theory and Society*. 9, (1), 131–75.

Latour, B. (1993) *We Have Never Been Modern*, translated by C. Porter, London: Harvester Wheatsheaf.

Law, J. (1992) 'Notes on the Theory of the Actor – Network Ordering, Strategy and Heterogeneity', *Systems Practice*, 5(4): 379–93.

Law, J. (1994) *Organizing Modernity*, Oxford: Blackwell.

LCVV (National Centre for Nursing and Care) (1997) website available at www.lcvv.nl/eng/organ

Lee, N. and Hassard, J. (1999) 'Organization Unbound: Actor Network Theory, Research Strategy and Institutional Flexibility', *Organization*, 6, (3), 391–404.

Levy, C. (1996) 'Introduction: Italian Regionalism in Context', in C. Levy (ed.) *Italian Regionalism: History, Identity and Politics*, Oxford: Berg, 1–29.

Lewis, J. (1989) 'Lone Parent Families: Politics and Economics', *Journal of Social Policy*, 18, (4), 595–600.

Lewis, J. (1992) 'Gender and the Development of Welfare Regimes', *Journal of European Social Policy*, 2, (3), 159–73.

Liaropoulos, L. and Kaitelidou, D. (1997) *Health Technology Assessment in Greece: Country Paper (2nd Draft)* Greece: Center for Health Services Management and Evaluation, University of Athens, October.

Liaropoulos, L. and Tragakes, E. (1998) 'Public/Private Financing in the Greek Health Care System: Implications for Equity', *Health Policy*, 43, 153–69.

Light, D. (1995) 'Countervailing Powers: A Framework for Professions in Transition', in T. Johnson, G. Larkin and M. Saks (eds) *Health Professions and the State in Europe*, London: Routledge, 25–41.

Light, D. (1997) 'From Managed Competition to Managed Cooperation: Theory and Lessons from the British Experience', *The Milbank Quarterly*, 75, (3), 297–341.

Light, D. (2000) 'Fostering a Justice-Based Health Care System', *Contemporary Sociology*, 29, (1), 62–74.

Lockwood, D. (1958) *The Blackcoated Worker*, London: George Allen & Unwin.

Lohmann, H. (2000) *Modernity Through Fit*, LBK Hamburg, Management Letter, ausgabe 2000/1, 4–7.

Lomas, J. Anderson, G. M. and Domnick-Pierre, K. (1989) 'Do Practice Guidelines Guide Practice? The Effect of a Consensus Statement on the Practice of Physicians', *The New England Journal of Medicine*, 321, 19, 1306–11.

Lowndes, V. (1996) 'Varieties of New Institutionalism: a Critical Appraisal', *Public Administration*, 74, 181–97.

Macdonald, K. M. (1995) *The Sociology of the Professions*, London: Sage.

Maclachlan, D. (1997) 'Specialist Training in Medicine in Germany', *BMJ*, 7100, vol. 315, Saturday 12 July, <www.bmj.com>

Macpherson, C. B. (1962) *The Political Theory of Possessive Individualism: Hobbes to Locke*, Oxford: Oxford University Press.

Maroudy, D. (1996) 'Training for Anaesthetic Nurses in France', *British Journal of Theatre Nursing*, 15, (10), 15–20.

Matsaganis, M. (1998) 'From the North Sea to the Mediterranean? Constraints to Health Care Reform in Greece', *International Journal of Health Care Services*, 28, (2), 333–48.

McGregor, S. (1999) 'Welfare, Neo-Liberalism and New Paternalism: Three Ways for Social Policy in Late Capitalist Societies', *Capital & Class*, 67, 91–118.

McKinlay, J. and Arches, J. (1985) 'Towards the Proletarianization of Physicians', *International Journal of Health Services* 15, 161–95.

Melia, K. (1987) *Learning and Working: the Occupational Socialization of Nurses*, London: Tavistock.

Meyer, J. W. and Rowan, B. (1991) 'Institutionalized Organizations: Formal Structure as Myth and Ceremony', in W. W. Powell and P. J. DiMaggio (eds) *The New Institutionalism in Organizational Analysis*, Chicago and London: The University of Chicago Press, 41–62.

Mohan, J. (1996) 'Accounts of the NHS Reforms: Macro-, Meso- and Micro-Level Perspectives', *Sociology of Health & Illness*, 18, (5), 675–98.

Moran, M. (1999) *Governing the Health Care State: A Comparative Study of the United Kingdom, the United States and Germany*, Manchester: Manchester University Press.

Moran, M. and Wood, B. (1993) *States, Regulation and the Medical Profession*, Buckingham: Open University Press.

Morgan, G. (1990) *Organizations in Society*, Basingstoke and London: Macmillan.

Morgan, P. and Potter, C. (1995) 'Professional Cultures and Paradigms of Quality in Health Care', in I. Kirkpatrick and M. Martinez Lucio (eds) *The Politics of Quality in the Public Sector*, London: Routledge, 166–89.

Mossialos, E. (1997) 'Citizens' Views on Health Care Systems in the 15 Member States of the European Union', *Health Economics*, 6, 109–16.

Mouzelis, N. P. (1986) *Politics in the Semi-Periphery: Early Parliamentarism in the Balkans and Latin America*, Basingstoke: Macmillan-now Palgrave.

Netherlands, Ministry of Education, Culture and Science, Ministry of Health, Welfare and Sport (1997) *Qualified for the Future: Coherent Training System for Nursing and Patient Care in The Netherlands: A Summary*, Zoetermeer/Rijswijk, May.

Newbacher, A. and Scheidges, R. (2000) 'Hier Herrscht Eine Mafia', *Der Spiegel*, 31 July, 49–50.

NHS Management Executive (1994) *Clinical Audit: 1994/95 and Beyond (EL[94]20)*, letter 28 February, Leeds: Department of Health.

Nikol, S. and Huehns, T. Y. (1995) 'Letters: Nurses Role is Narrowing in Germany', *BMJ*, 311, 873.

O'Connor, J. S. (1993) 'Gender, Class and Citizenship in Comparative Analysis of Welfare State Regimes: Theoretical and Methodological Issues', *British Journal of Sociology*, 44, (3), 501–18.

O'Connor, J. S. (1996) 'Trend Report: From Women in the Welfare State to Gendering Welfare State Regimes', *Current Sociology*, 44, (2), 1–124.

O'Dowd, A. (2002) 'Professional Regulation: Meet the Man with the Plan', *Nursing Times*, 98, (13), 11–12.

OECD (Organisation for Economic Cooperation and Development) (1992) *The Reform of Health Care: A Comparative Analysis of Seven OECD Countries*, Paris: OECD.

OECD (1994) *The Reform of Health Care Systems: A Review of Seventeen OECD Countries*, Paris: OECD.

OECD (2000) *OECD Health Data 2000: A Comparative Analysis of 29 Countries*, Paris: OECD/CREDES.

OECD (2002) *OECD in Figures: Statistics on the Member Countries*, Paris: OECD, available at www1.oecd.org/publications/e-book/0102071e.pdf

Offe, C. (1984) *Contradictions of the Welfare State*, London: Hutchinson.

Orloff, A. S. (1993) 'Gender and the Social Rights of Citizenship: the Comparative Analysis of Gender Relations and Welfare States', *American Sociological Review*, 58, 303–28.

Osborne, T. and Gaebler, D. (1992) *Reinventing Government*, Reading, MA: Addison-Wesley.

Oud, N. E. (1997) 'Nursing Research in The Netherlands 1997', Workgroup of European Nurse Researchers (WENR) available at www.wenr/org/view_categories.php?nCatId=17

Pacitti, D. (2002) *Italy and its Discontents: Family, Civil Society, State 1980–2001*–Paul Ginsborg, book review Allen Lane/Penguin Press, *Times Higher Educational Supplement*, 27 September, 38.

Paquier, M. P. (1993) 'France', in S. Quinn and S. Russell (eds) *Nursing: The European Dimension*, London: Scutari Press, 77–84.

Parker, D. and Lawton, R. (2000) 'Judging the Use of Clinical Protocols by Fellow Professionals', *Social Science & Medicine*, 51, 669–77.

Paul, C. and Reeves, J. S. (1995) 'An Overview of the Nursing Process', in J. B. George (ed.) *Nursing Theories: The Base for Professional Nursing Practice* (4th edn), London: Prentice Hall International (UK), 15–31.

Perleth, M. and Busse, R. (1998) *The German Healthcare System*, Hanover Medical School, Germany, available at http://www.epi.mh-hannover.de/

Petmesidou, M. (1996) 'Social Protection in Greece: A Brief Glimpse of a Welfare State', *Social Policy and Administration*, 30, (4), 324–47.

Piattoni, S. (1998) '"Virtuous Clientelism": The Southern Question Resolved?', in J. Schneider (ed.) *Italy's 'Southern Question': Orientalism in One Country*, Oxford: Berg, 225–44.

Pickvance, C. J. (1999) 'Democratisation and the Decline of Social Movements: The Effects of Regime Change on Collective Action in Eastern Europe and Latin America', *Sociology*, 33, (2), 353–72.

Pollitt, C. (2001) 'Convergence: The Useful Myth', *Public Administration*, 79, (4), 933–47.

Pollitt, C. and Bouckaert, G. (2000) *Public Management Reform: a Comparative Analysis*, Oxford: Oxford University Press.

Powell, W. W. (1991) '"Neither Market nor Hierarchy" Network Forms of Organization', in G. Thomspon, J. Frances, R. Levačić and J. Mitchell (eds) *Markets, Hierarchies and Networks: The Coordination of Social Life*, London: Sage, 265–76.

Powell, W. W. and DiMaggio, P. J. (eds) (1991) *The New Institutionalism in Organizational Analysis*, Chicago and London: University of Chicago Press.

Power, M. (1994) *The Audit Explosion*, London: Demos.

Power, M. (1997) *The Audit Society: The Rituals of Verification*, Oxford: Oxford University Press.

Pratschke, J. (2000) 'The Work Grievances of Hospital Nurses in Ireland and Southern Italy', paper presented at the *International Labour Process Conference*, University of Strathclyde, Glasgow.

Putnam, R. D. (1993) *Making Democracy Work: Civic Traditions in Modern Italy*, Princeton, NJ: Princeton University Press.

Quinn, S. and Russell, S. (1993) *Nursing: The European Dimension*, London: Scutari Press.

Ranade, W. (1997) *A Future for the NHS? Health Care for the Millennium* (2nd edn), London and New York: Longman.

Ranade, W. (1998) 'Introduction' in W. Ranade (ed.) *Markets and Health Care: A Comparative Analysis*, London: Longman, 1–16.

Reerink, E. (1990) 'Improving the Quality of Hospital Services in The Netherlands: the Role of the CBO', *Quality Assurance in Health Care*, 2, (1), 13–19.

Rehnberg, C. (1997) 'Sweden', in C. Ham (ed.) *Health Care Reform: Learning from International Experience*, Buckingham: Open University Press, 64–86.

Reuters (1999) 'Poland: Focus – Polish Hospital Row Takes Turn for the Worse', Warsaw, 1 January, accessed at www.centraleurope.com.

Richard, S. and Schönbach, K-H. (1996) 'German Sickness Funds Under Fixed Budgets', in F. W. Schwarz, H. Glennester and R.B. Saltman (eds) *Fixing Health Budgets: Experiences from Europe and North America*, Chichester: Wiley, 187–201.

Ritzer, G. (1996) *The McDonaldization of Society* (revised edn), London: Pine Forge Press.

Rosenthal, M. M. (1992) 'Medical Discipline in Cross-Cultural Perspective: the United States, Britain and Sweden', in R. Dingwall and Paul Fenn (eds) *Quality and Regulation in Health Care: International Experiences*, London: Routledge, 26–50.

Rosenthal, M. M. (2002) '"Medical Professional Autonomy in an Era of Accountability and Regulation": Voices of Doctors Under Siege', in M. Dent and S. Whitehead (eds) *Managing Professional Identities: Knowledge, Performativity and the 'New' Professional*, London: Routledge, 61–80.

Sackett, D. L. Rosenberg, W. M. C. Gray, J. A. M. Haynes, R. B. and Richardson, W. S. (1996) 'Evidence-based medicine: What It Is and What It Isn't', *BMJ*, 13 January, 71–2.

Sackett, D. L. and Wennberg, J. E. (1997) 'Choosing the Best Research Design for Each Question', editorial, 20/27 December *BMJ*, 315 (7123).

Sahlin-Andersson, K. (1994) 'Group Identities as the Building Blocks of Organisations: a Story About Nurses' Daily Work', *Scandinavian Journal of Management*, 10, (2), 131–45.

Sainsbury, D. (1994) 'Introduction', in D. Sainsbury (ed.) *Gendering Welfare States*, London: Sage, 1–7.

Saltman, R. B. (1990) 'Competition and Reform in the Swedish Health System', *The Milbank Quarterly*, 68, (4), 597–618.

Saltman, R. B. (1997) 'Convergence versus Social Embeddedness: Debating the Future Direction of Health Care Systems', *European Journal of Public Health*, 7, 449–53.

Saltman, R. B. and von Otter, C. (1992) *Planned Markets and Public Competition: Strategic Reforms in Northern European Health Systems*, Buckingham: Open University Press.

Salvage, J. and Heijnen, S. (1997) 'Nursing and Midwifery in Europe', in J. Salvage and S. Heijnen (eds) *Nursing in Europe: A Resource for Better Health*, WHO Regional Publications, European Series, No. 74, Copenhagen: World Health Organization, Regional Office for Europe, 21–126.

Samatas, M. (1993) 'Debureaucratization Failure in Post-Dictatorial Greece: a Socio-Political Control Approach', *Journal of Modern Greek Studies*, 11, (2), 187–217.

Saraceno, C. and Negri, N. (1994) 'The Changing Italian Welfare State', *Journal of European Social Policy*, 4, (1), 19–34.

Schepers, R. M. and Casparie, R. M. J. (1997) 'Continuity or Discontinuity in the Self-Regulation of the Belgian and Dutch Medical Professions', *Sociology of Health and Illness*, 19, (5), 580–600.

Schut, F. T. (1995) *Competition in the Dutch Health Care Sector*, Den Haag: Cip-Gegevens Koninklijke Biblitheek.

Schwartz, F. W. and Busse, R. (1997) 'Germany', in C. Ham (ed.) *Health Care Reform: Learning from International Experience*, Buckingham: Open University Press, 104–118.

Scott, W. R., Ruef, M., Mendel, P. J. and Caronna, C. A. (2000) *Institutional Change and Healthcare Organizations: From Professional Dominance to Managed Care*, Chicago and London: University of Chicago Press.

Secretary of State for Health (1999) *The New NHS: Modern – Dependable*, London: The Stationary Office.

Selznick, P. (1949) *TVA and the Grass Roots*, Berkeley, University of California Press.

Sewell, G. and Wilkinson, B. (1992) 'Someone to Watch Over Me: Surveillance, Discipline, and the Just-In-Time Labour Process', *Sociology*, 26, (2), 271–91.

Siegrist, H. (1990) 'Professionalization as a Process: Patterns, Progression and Discontinuity', in M. Burrage and R. Torstendahl (eds) *Professions in Theory and History*, London: Sage, 177–202.

Sissouras, A., Karokis, A. and Mossialos, E. (1994) '11. Greece', in OECD, *The Reform of Health Care Systems: a Review of Seventeen OECD Countries*, Paris: OECD.

Sissouras, A., Karokis, A. and Mossialos, E. (1999) 'Health Care and Cost Containment in Greece', in E. Mossialos and J. Le Grand (eds) *Health Care and Cost Containment in the European Union'*, Aldershot: Ashgate, 341–400.

Smith, M. (1988) 'Some Historical Problems of Corporatist Developments in the Netherlands', in A. Cox and N. O'Sullivan (eds) *The Corporate State: Corporatism and the State Tradition in Western Europe*, Aldershot: Edward Elger, 170–97.

Sobczak, A. (1996) *Changes in the Polish Health Care System in the 1990–95 Transition Period*, Working Papers No. 50. Warsaw: Institute of Finance

Sobczak, A. (1998) *Universal Health Insurance in Poland*, Working Papers No. 56. Warsaw: Institute of Finance.

Spence, R. (1996) 'Italy', in A. Wall (ed.) *Health Care Systems in Liberal Democracies*, London: Routledge, 47–75.

Stallknecht, K. (1992) 'Nursing in Europe', in T. Richards (ed.) *Medicine in Europe*, London: *British Medical Journal*: 59–64.

Standing, G. (1996) 'Social Protection in Central and Eastern Europe: a Tale of Slipping Anchors and Torn Safety Nets', in G. Esping-Andersen (ed.) *Welfare States in Transition: National Adaptations in Global Economies*, London: Sage, 225–55.

Stecka-Feffer, H. (1996) 'A Short Outline of the History of Nursing Training in Poland', *International History of Nursing Journal*, 1, (4), 72–6.

Stevens, F. (2001) 'The Convergence and Divergence of Modern Health Care Systems', in W. C. Cockerham (ed.) *The Blackwell Companion to Medical Sociology*, Oxford: Blackwell, 159–76.

Strauss, A., Fagerhaugh, S., Suczek, B. and Wiener, C. (1982) 'Sentimental Work in the Technologized Hospital', *Sociology of Health & Illness*, 4, (3), 257–78.

Strauss, A., Fagerhaugh, S., Suczek, B. and Wiener, C. (1985) *Social Organization of Medical Work*, Chicago and London: University of Chicago Press.

TA NEA [The Hours] (1998) Κατεβάζουν τα ρολά οι γιατοί, 23 Δεκεμβρίου: 16.

Thompson, P. (1990) 'Crawling from the Wreckage: the Labour Process and the Politics of Production', in D. Knights and H. Willmott (eds) *Labour Process Theory*, London: Macmillan, 95–124.

Trifiletti, R. (1999) 'Southern European Welfare Regimes and the Worsening Position of Women', *Journal of European Social Policy*, 9, (1), 49–64.

Vail, M. I. (1999) 'The Better Part of Valour: The Politics of French Welfare Regime', *Journal of European Health Policy*, 9, (4), 3100–29.

van de Ven, W. (1997) 'The Netherlands', in C. Ham (ed.) *Health Care Reform: Learning from International Experience*, Buckingham: Open University Press: 87–103.

van de Ven, W. P. M. M. and van Vliet, R. C. J. A. (1997) 'How can we Prevent Cream Skimming in a Competitive Health Insurance Market? The Greatest Challenge for the 90s', in P. Zweifel and H. E. Frech (eds) *Health Economic Worldwide*, Dordrecht: Kluwer, 23–46.

van der Grintern, T. E. D. and Kasdorp, J. P. (1999) 'Choices in Dutch Health Care: Mixing Strategies and Responsibilities', *Health Policy*, 50, 105–22.

VOMIL (Ministry of Public Health and Environment) (1974) *Memorandum on the Structure of Health Care*, Leidschendam: Ministry of Public Health and Environment.

Walby, S. and Greenwell, J. with L. Mackay and K. Soothill (1994) *Medicine and Nursing: Professions in a Changing Health Service*, London: Sage.

Walshe, K. (2002) 'The Rise of Regulation in the NHS', *BMJ*, 324, 967–70.

Wanless. D. (Chair) (2001) *Securing Our Future: Taking a Long-Term Review* (Wanless Report), London: HM Treasury, available at www.hmtreasury.gov.uk/ Consultations and Legislation/wanless/consult wanless final.cfm

Wasem, J. (1997) 'Health Care Reform in the Federal Republic of Germany: The New and Old Länder', in C. Altenstetter and J.W. Björkman (eds) *Health Policy Reform, National Variations and Globalization*, Basingstoke: Macmillan, 161–74.

Weick, K. E. (1976) 'Educational Organizations as Loosely Coupled Systems', *Administrative Science Quarterly*, 21, 1–19.

Whitehead, M., Gustafsson, R. A. and Diderichsen, F. (1997) 'Why is Sweden Rethinking its NHS Style Reforms?' *BMJ*, 315, 935–9.

Whitehead, S. (2002) *Men and Masculinities*, Cambridge: Polity.

WHO (World Health Organization) (1985) *Targets for Health for All*, Regional Office for Europe, Copenhagen: WHO.

WHO (1994) *The Netherlands: Nursing and Midwifery Profile*, December Copenhagen: World Health Organization.

WHO (1996) *Health Care Systems in Transition: Sweden*, Copenhagen (preliminary version), Regional Office for Europe.

WHO (2000a) *United Kingdom: Nursing and Midwifery Profile*, unedited update, May, Copenhagen, Denmark: World Health Organization, Regional Office for Europe, available at http://www.wh.dk/Nursing/welcome.htm

WHO (2000b) *France: Nursing and Midwifery Profile*, unedited update – May, Copenhagen, Denmark: World Health Organization, Regional Office for Europe, available at http://www.wh.dk/Nursing/welcome.htm

WHO (2000c) *Sweden: Nursing and Midwifery Profile*, Copenhagen: World Health Organization, available at www.who.dk/nursing.htm

WHO (2000d) *Germany: Nursing and Midwifery Profile*, Copenhagen: World Health Organization, available at www.who.dk/nursing.htm

WHO (2001) *Health For All Database*, Copenhagen: WHO Regional Office for Europe.

WHO Statistics (2002) *WHO Estimates of Health Personnel*, World Health Organization, available at www3.who.int/whois/health_personnel/health-personnel.cfm.

Wiley, M. M. (1998) 'Financing Operating Costs for Acute Hospital Services', in R. B. Saltman, J. Figueras and C. Sakellarides (eds) *Critical Challenges for Health Care Reform in Europe*, Buckingham: Open University Press, 218–35.

Williams, K. (1980) 'From Sarah Gamp to Florence Nightingale: a Critical Study of Hospital Nursing Systems from 1840–1897', in C. Davies (ed.) *Rewriting Nursing History*, London: Croom Helm, 41–75.

Williamson, O. E. (1975) *Markets and Hierarchies: Analysis and Antitrust Implications*, New York: Free Press.

Wilsford, D. (1991) *Doctors and the State: The Politics of Health Care in France and the US*, Durham and London: Duke University Press.

Wilsford, D. (1994) 'Path Dependency, or Why History Makes It Difficult but Not Impossible to Reform Health Care Systems in a Big Way', *Journal of Public Policy*, 14, (3), 251–83.

Wilsford, D. (1995) 'States Facing Interests: Struggles Over Health Care Policy in Advanced Industrial Democracies', *Journal of Health Politics, Policy and Law*, 20, (3), 571–614.

Witz, A. (1992) *Professions and Patriarchy*, London: Routledge.

Witz, A. (1995) 'The Challenge of Nursing', in J. Gabe, D. Kelleher and G. Williams (eds) *Challenging Medicine*, London: Routledge, 23–45.

Subject Index

Author Index